DR. SEBI

CURE FOR HERPES

The Real Guide on How to Naturally Cure and Treat Herpes Virus and get Benefits Through Dr. Sebi Alkaline Diet

BY

ALFRED BEGUM

Copyright 2020 by Alfred Begum

All rights reserved.

This document is geared towards providing exact and reliable information with regards to the topic and issue covered. The publication is sold with the idea that the publisher is not required to render accounting, officially permitted, or otherwise, qualified services. If advice is necessary, legal or professional, a practiced individual in the profession should be ordered.

-From a Declaration of Principles which was accepted and approved equally by a Committee of the American Bar Association and a Committee of Publishers and Associations.

In no way is it legal to reproduce, duplicate, or transmit any part of this document in either electronic means or in printed format. Recording of this publication is strictly prohibited and any storage of this document is not allowed unless with written permission from the publisher. All rights reserved.

The information provided herein is stated to be truthful and consistent, in that any liability, in terms of inattention or otherwise, by any usage or abuse of any policies, processes, or directions contained within is the solitary and utter responsibility of the recipient reader. Under no circumstances will any legal responsibility or blame be held against the publisher for any reparation, damages, or monetary loss due to the information herein, either directly or indirectly.

Respective authors own all copyrights not held by the publisher.

The information herein is offered for informational purposes solely, and is universal as so. The presentation of the information is without contract or any type of guarantee assurance.

The trademarks that are used are without any consent, and the publication of the trademark is without permission or backing by the trademark owner. All trademarks and brands within this book are for clarifying purposes only and are the owned by the owners themselves, not affiliated with this document.

Table of Contents

Introduction.

Chapter one: What is herpes virus and what should you know?.

Chapter two: The alkaline diet

Chapter three: advantages of the diet and tips for starting.

Chapter four: Some disease and Dr sebi herbal cure.

Chapter five: Alkaline diet

Chapter Six: Who is Dr. Sebi

Chapter seven: The Dr. Sebi Herpes cure.

Chapter eight: Fasting and Dr. Sebi diet

Conclusion.

Introduction

Unfortunately, Herpes has been stigmatized as probably one of the worst things that could happen to you the truth however is that it can happen to anyone. The media and pop culture mock carriers of this virus. Out of fear of being ostracized, people with genital herpes also fear letting even close friends and relatives hear about their disease. Medical practitioners have also been known to make outrageous statements such as "for the rest of your life, you must take this costly anti-retroviral drug, and You should never have sex again"! This is unfortunate, because the fact remains that herpes is a condition that requires much more education that is greatly overlooked. It's rubbish to believe that you'd never have sex again or that you must be stuck with using an Anti Retroviral drug for years. One of the most prevalent diseases in the world is HSV-1 (common oral herpes) and HSV-2 (genital herpes), and it's not something to worry over. Moreover, in the form of a specific and natural strategy, there is a herpes treatment that can be applied and it will not only improve the quality of your life, but it will also stop breakouts from ever happening again. We will explore how to handle the virus functions in this book, some of the popular strategies for coping with herpes, and the natural preventive approach we think will significantly minimize the amount of discomfort caused by the virus. Yeah, it is annoying to have herpes, but a diagnosis is not the end of the universe. Currently, it is difficult to find someone who is NOT afflicted with any type of HSV. Don't believe the herpes propaganda. Instead, get the truth on the condition and establish a successful plan to eradicate it.

Dr. Sebi thought that the Western response to the epidemic was inadequate. He assumed the illness was caused by acidity and mucus that bred bacteria and viruses. A major dietary theory is that only in acidic environments can disease occur. The aim of the diet is to preserve alkaline conditions in the body in order to prevent or eradicate the disease.

Botanical medications that help to detoxify the body are provided on the official diet website. The Commission reports that the claims were not studied by the Food and Drug Administration (FDA).

Doctor Sebi Diet-is this safe for you?

Analysis shows, however that well-being would be enhanced by a diet based on vegetables. In the following segment, there are other problems that we will discuss. Other advantages of herbal diets for health can include:

1. Weight loss -a vegan diet led to greater weight loss than other, less restrictive diets in the 2015 study. The participants lost up to 7.5 percent of their body weight on a vegan diet after six months.

2. Appetite management-A 2016 study of young male participants found that they felt more comfortable and healthier after eating a meal containing peas and beans than after a meal containing beef.

3. Modification of microbiome-the term 'microbiome' usually refers to intestinal microorganisms. In 2019, a research study found that a plant-based diet could favorably alter the microbiome and lead to a lower risk of disease. To confirm this however, further work will be needed.

4.   A plant-based diet report in 2017 showed that the risk for coronary heart disease could be decreased by 40 percent and the chance of developing metabolic syndrome and type 2 diabetes by nearly half.

The lifestyle of Dr. Sebi promotes individuals to eat raw ingredients and eliminates processed goods. A research in 2017 found that a reduction in processed food intake would improve the average dietary quality of the U.S. diet. The diet of Dr. Sebi is strict and does not contain sufficient significant nutrients that are not clearly listed on the website of the diet. If a person follows a diet, a healthcare professional who can advise on suitable supplements may support him or her.

Chapter one: What is herpes virus and what should you know?

More generally referred to as herpes, herpes simplex viruses are classified into two types: type 1 herpes (HSV-1, or oral herpes) and type 2 herpes (HSV-2, or genital herpes). Herpes type 1 most often triggers sores (sometimes referred to as fever blisters or cold sores) across the mouth and lips. HSV-1 can cause genital herpes, but herpes type 2 causes the majority of cases of genital herpes. In HSV-2, sores around the genitals or rectum can occur in the infected person. While in other areas, HSV-2 sores can occur, these sores are typically located below the waist.

However, in order to induce inflammation in or near the genital region (genital herpes), HSV-1 can also be spread by oral-genital contact. HSV-2 is almost entirely spread during sex by genital-to-genital contact, triggering genital or anal area (genital herpes) infection. Both oral herpes and genital herpes infections are often asymptomatic or unrecognized, but at the site of diagnosis, they can cause signs of painful blisters or ulcers varying from mild to serious.

Type-1 herpes simplex virus (HSV-1)

HSV-1 is an extremely infectious virus that is widespread and endemic worldwide. During puberty, most HSV-1 diseases are acquired, and infection is permanent. Oral herpes (infections in or near the mouth, also referred to as orolabial, oral-labial or oral-facial herpes) is the vast majority of HSV-1 infections, although a proportion of HSV-1 infections are genital herpes (infections in the genital or anal area).

Symptoms and signs

The infection of oral herpes is often asymptomatic, and most people with HSV-1 infection do not know they are sick. Oral herpes symptoms include painful blisters in or near the mouth or raw sores called ulcers. Sores on the lips are generally referred to as "cold sores." Before the emergence of sores, affected individuals will frequently feel a tingling, scratching or burning feeling around their mouth. The blisters or ulcers will regularly recur after initial infection. The frequency of recurrences ranges from individual to individual. HSV-1-caused genital herpes may be asymptomatic or have minor signs that go unrecognized. If signs do appear, 1 or more genital or anal blisters or ulcers are described by genital herpes. Symptoms may recur after an initial episode of genital herpes, which can be serious. Unlike genital herpes caused by herpes simplex virus type 2 (HSV-2; see below), however, genital herpes caused by HSV-1 usually does not recur frequently.

The Transmission

In order to induce oral herpes infection, HSV-1 is spread primarily by oral-to-oral contact, by interaction with the HSV-1 virus in the sores, saliva, and surfaces in or near the mouth. HSV-1 can however, also be spread by oral-genital contact to the genital region to induce genital herpes. HSV-1 may be spread from surfaces of the oral or skin that look natural even where no signs are present. The biggest chance of transmitting, however, is when active sores are present. It is doubtful that persons who currently have HSV-1 oral herpes infection would eventually become infected with HSV-1 in the genital region. HSV-1 infection can in extreme cases, be transferred from a mother with genital HSV-1 infection to her child to induce neonatal herpes during childbirth (see below).

Complications

Extreme illness: HSV-1 may have more severe symptoms and more frequent recurrences in immunocompromised patients, such as those with advanced HIV infection. More significant complications, such as encephalitis (brain infection) or keratitis (eye infection), can often occasionally arise from HSV-1 infection.

Neonatal herpes: When a child is exposed to HSV (HSV-1 or HSV-2) in the genital tract during birth, neonatal herpes can occur. Neonatal herpes is rare, occurring worldwide in an estimated 10 out of every 100,000 births, but it is a dangerous disease that can lead to severe neurological damage or death. Women who have genital herpes have a very low chance of passing HSV to their children before they become pregnant. When a mother first acquires HSV infection in late pregnancy, the risk for neonatal herpes is greater. Partially because the levels of HSV in the genital tract are higher early in infection.

Psychosocial impact: Persistent oral herpes symptoms can be painful and can lead to some social isolation and psychological trauma. These variables may have an important effect on the quality of life and sexual experiences with genital herpes. In time, however most individuals with any form of herpes adapt to dealing with the infection.

Treatment: The most effective drugs available for people afflicted with HSV are antiviral medications such as acyclovir, famciclovir, and valacyclovir. These can help decrease the severity and duration of symptoms, but the infection can not be healed medically.

WHO general recommendations for the treatment of Simplex Virus Genital Herpes

<u>Prevention</u>

During an epidemic of symptomatic oral herpes, HSV-1 is most infectious, but may also be spread where no signs are felt or noticeable. People with active oral herpes symptoms should avoid making oral contact with others and exchanging saliva-contact items. To stop spreading herpes to a sexual partner's anus, they should also abstain from oral sex. Individuals with signs of genital herpes and having all of the symptoms should abstain from sexual intercourse. People who are still infected with HSV-1 are not at risk of developing it again, but they are also at risk of genital infection with herpes simplex virus type 2 (HSV-2). In order to avoid the transmission of genital herpes, the effective and proper use of condoms will help. However, condoms can only reduce the risk of infection, and in places not protected by condoms, outbreaks of genital herpes can occur. People who are still infected with HSV-1 are not at risk of getting it again, but they are also at risk of getting genital HSV-2 infection. Pregnant women with genital herpes signs should be advised by their health care providers. It is especially necessary for women in late pregnancy to avoid the development of a new genital herpes infection, as this is when the risk of neonatal herpes is highest. In order to develop more efficient prevention strategies against HSV infection, such as vaccines, more research is ongoing. Currently, multiple candidate HSV vaccines are being tested.

Herpes simplex virus type 2 (HSV-2)

Infection with HSV-2 is widespread worldwide and is almost entirely transmitted sexually, causing genital herpes. The major cause of genital herpes, which can also be caused by the type 1 herpes simplex virus (HSV-1), is HSV-2. HSV-2 infection is lifelong and incurable.

Scope of the subject

HSV-2-induced genital herpes is a global problem, with an estimated 491 million (13 percent) individuals aged 15 to 49 years worldwide living with the infection in 2016. More women than men are infected with HSV-2; 313 million females and 178 million males were estimated to be living with the infection in 2016. This is because HSV sexual transmission is more effective from male to female than from female to male. It has been estimated that the prevalence of HSV-2 infection is highest in Africa (44% in women and 25% in men), followed by the Americas (24% in women and 12% in men). Prevalence has also been shown to increase with age, although adolescents were the largest number of people newly infected.

Symptoms and signs

Infections with genital herpes often have no symptoms or mild symptoms that go unrecognized. The majority of people infected are unaware that they have the infection. About 10-20 percent of individuals with HSV-2 infection typically report a prior diagnosis of genital herpes. Clinical trials that closely follow individuals for new infections, however, show that up to a third of people with new infections may have symptoms. When symptoms do happen, one or more genital or anal blisters or open sores called ulcers are characterized by genital herpes. The symptoms of new genital herpes infections often include fever, body aches, and swollen lymph nodes, in addition to genital ulcers. Recurrent symptoms are common but often less severe than the first outbreak after an initial genital herpes infection with HSV-2. Over time, the frequency of outbreaks tends to decline, but may occur for many years. HSV-2 infected individuals may experience sensations of mild tingling or shooting pain in the legs, hips, and buttocks before genital ulcers appear.

Transmission

HSV-2 is mainly transmitted during sex, through contact with someone infected with the virus's genital surfaces, skin, sores or fluids. In the genital or anal area, HSV-2 may be transmitted from the skin that looks normal and is often transmitted in the absence of symptoms. HSV-2 infection can be transmitted from a mother to her infant during delivery to cause neonatal herpes in rare circumstances (see below).

Possible complications

HSV-2 as well as HIV: It has been demonstrated that HSV-2 and HIV influence each other. Infection with HSV-2 increases the risk of acquiring a new HIV infection by about three-fold. In fact, individuals with both HIV and HSV-2 disease are more likely to spread HIV to others. In people living with HIV, HSV-2 is among the most common infections, occurring in 60-90 percent of people infected with HIV. HSV-2 infection can have a more severe presentation and more frequent recurrences in people living with HIV (and other immunocompromised individuals). HSV-2 may lead to more severe but rare complications in advanced HIV disease, such as meningoencephalitis, oesophagitis, hepatitis, pneumonitis, retinal necrosis or disseminated infection.

Neonatal herpes: When an infant is exposed to HSV (HSV-2 or HSV-1) in the genital tract during delivery, neonatal herpes can occur. Neonatal herpes is rare, occurring worldwide in an estimated 10 out of every

100,000 births, but it is a dangerous disease that can lead to severe neurological damage or death. Women who have genital herpes have a very low chance of passing HSV to their children before they become pregnant. When a mother acquires HSV infection for the first time in late pregnancy, the risk for neonatal herpes is greatest, partly because the levels of HSV in the genital tract are highest early in infection.

Psychosocial influence: Recurrent genital herpes symptoms may be painful and social stigma and psychological distress may result from the infection. Such variables can have a significant impact on the quality of life and sexual relations. However most individuals with herpes adjust to living with the infection in time.

<u>Therapy</u>

The most effective medications available for people infected with HSV include antivirals such as acyclovir, famciclovir, and valacyclovir. These can help decrease the severity and duration of symptoms, but the infection can not be healed.

WHO guidelines for the treatment of Simplex Virus Genital Herpes

<u>Prevention</u>

Individuals with genital HSV infection while experiencing symptoms of genital herpes should abstain from sexual activity. During an outbreak of sores, HSV-2 is the most contagious, but can also be transmitted when no symptoms are felt or visible. People with symptoms suggestive of genital HSV infection should also receive HIV testing, and more focused HIV prevention efforts, such as pre-exposure prophylaxis, could benefit those in settings or populations with high HIV incidence. Consistent and correct condom use can help to reduce the risk of genital herpes spreading. Condoms provide only partial protection, however as HSV can be found in areas not covered by a condom. In addition to HIV and human papillomavirus (HPV), medical male circumcision can provide males with life-long partial HSV-2 protection. Pregnant women with genital herpes signs should be advised by their health care providers. It is especially necessary for women in late pregnancy to avoid the development of a new genital herpes infection, as this is when the risk of neonatal herpes is highest. Further research is underway to develop more effective methods of prevention against HSV infection, such as vaccines or topical microbicides (compounds that can be applied to protect against sexually transmitted infections inside the vagina or rectum).

Herpes response from the WHO (HSV-1 and HSV-2)

Improved access to antiviral medications and increased HIV prevention efforts for those with genital HSV symptoms are needed globally, as well as increasing awareness about HSV infection and its symptoms. In addition, there is a need to develop better treatment and prevention interventions, especially HSV vaccines. The WHO and its collaborators are working to promote research and create novel methods for genital and neonatal HSV-1 and HSV-2 infection prevention and management. The development of HSV vaccines and topical microbicides involves such research. Several vaccines and microbicides for candidates are currently being studied.

Chapter two: The alkaline diet

What is Dr. sebi diet and how does it work?

Dr. Sebi thought that the Western response to the epidemic was inadequate. He assumed the illness was caused by acidity and mucus that bred bacteria and viruses. A major dietary theory is that only in acidic environments can disease occur. The aim of the diet is to preserve alkaline conditions in the body in order to prevent or eradicate the disease. Botanical medications that help to detoxify the body are provided on the official diet website. Any literature supporting its protection benefit statements is not related to the site. The Commission reports that the claims were not studied by the Food and Drug Administration (FDA). The developers realize that they are not trained professionals and do not wish to make professional suggestions.

Methodology

Sometimes a single step will lead you to a state you've never dreamed of. The fight that eventually leads to a healthy lifestyle would be to go on an alkaline diet. An alkaline diet is an assumption that an alkaline deposit or ash is left behind in the body by such things, such as fruit, fruits, roots, and legumes. The primary components of rock, such as calcium, magnesium, titanium, zinc and copper, protect the body. An alkaline diet is the best preventive method for preventing chronic illnesses such as asthma, malnutrition, fatigue, and even cancer.

Here are few methods to successfully embrace the alkaline diet:

Drink water - Water is perhaps the most essential (after oxygen) resource for our body. As the water content influences the composition of the body, hydration of the body is essential. To preserve the body well hydrated (filtered to cleaned), drink about 8-10 glasses of water.

Our body also helps to regulate the acid and alkaline content by eliminating acidic beverages such as tea, coffee, or soda. In carbonated beverages, there is no reason to blink, as the body avoids carbon dioxide as waste!

Breathe - Oxygen is the clarification of how our body functions, and it can function faster if you supply the body with enough oxygen. Sit down and enjoy deep breathing for two to five minutes. Nothing is simpler than being able to do yoga.

The body has not been conditioned to ingest those chemicals, because the body then consumes or preserves them as fat, and they do not harm the liver. Avoid food with preservatives and food colors. Acids are formed by chemicals, so that the body neutralizes them either by producing cholesterol or by blanching iron from the RBCs (leading to anemia) or by removing calcium from the bones (osteoporosis).

Avoid artificial flavorings - These sweeteners are potentially toxic to the body, tending to be rich in low fat. Furthermore, Saccharin, a key ingredient in sweeteners, allows cancer to do any damage to the cells by removing these acids and even reversing the decomposition process. Therefore, stay away from these things. Go for less nutritious food, a good one anyway.

Exercise- There is also a match between the alkaline and acidic elements. This is not simply a case of alkaline milk being brought in. Natural bodywork is also influenced by a little acid (because of muscles).

By eating salads or soaked nuts, fulfill the desires for a snack - we also consume a little fast food while we are thirsty. Build a tradition of eating almonds or fresh vegetables, sometimes walnuts.

Eat the correct combination of food - When digested, the fats and proteins of carbohydrates require a special environment. And don't eat all at once. Test and correctly match the food composition to create the optimum mix of all the nutrients that you absorb.

Using green powder as an alternative to food - This helps to enhance the body's alkaline consistency.

Nice night - Attempt to escape the agony. Our mind controls the digestive system, and you can only know that it operates correctly when in a calm, centered state. Relax and stay safe, then,

Is this particular diet safe for you?

Analysis shows, however a diet would enhance that well-being based on vegetables. In the following segment, there are other problems that we will discuss. Other advantages of herbal diets for health can include:

Weight loss -a vegan diet led to greater weight loss than other, less restrictive diets in the 2015 study. The participants lost up to 7.5 percent of their body weight on a vegan diet after six months.

Appetite management-A 2016 study of young male participants found that they felt more comfortable and healthier after eating a meal containing peas and beans than after a meal containing beef.

Modification of microbiome-the term 'microbiome' usually refers to intestinal microorganisms. In 2019, a research study found that a plant-based diet could favorably alter the microbiome and lead to a lower risk of disease. To confirm this however, further work will be needed.

A plant-based diet report in 2017 showed that the risk for coronary heart disease could be decreased by 40 percent and the chance of developing metabolic syndrome and type 2 diabetes by nearly half. The lifestyle of Dr. Sebi promotes individuals to eat raw ingredients and eliminates processed goods. Research in 2017 found that a reduction in processed food intake would improve the U.S. diet's average dietary quality. Dr. Sebi's diet is strict and does not contain sufficient significant nutrients that are not clearly listed on the diet's website. If a person follows a diet, a healthcare professional who can advise on suitable supplements may support him or her.

Self-cleansing herbs and revitalizing the body

Detoxification or detox depends on the sort of fasting you choose and frankly, if you eat any of the cleansing herbs during your fasting time, it would serve you well. However, if you want to fast for a week then you can only drink water and the cleansing herbs in a tea during the week and nothing else should be eaten.

List & Use

1. Cascara sagrada is a shrub herb, which most people only recognize as a "dietary supplement," which was licensed to market as over the counter products in pharmacies. In 2002, however the FDA reported that it did not meet the requirements to be advertised as over the counter drugs (OTC) or prescription drugs. Before then the Cascara Sagrada dietary supplement or bark was used as a constipation purgative. The fact that it is a less bitter extract that can also be used as a flavoring agent is one sweet thing about this shrub.

2. The Rhubarb Root is the Rhubarb plant's root and underground stem (i.e., rhizome). The root of this plant has been used as a medicine for the treatment of digestive tract disease by traditional Chinese people, including stomach pain, constipation, menstrual cramps (dysmenorrhea), diarrhea, pancreatic swelling, etc. This plant's stems are often used as a flavoring agent and are primarily used to make tar and serve as great recipes. Studies also shown that it is a potent laxative that has the potential to minimize swelling, relieve cold sores and enhance the tone and wellbeing of the digestive tract, cleans heavy metal and toxic bacteria, improve the general movement of the intestines and even decrease the amount of cholesterol because of the chemicals found in Rhubarb root such as fiber.

3. It is a flowering plant/shrub from the daisy family and native to Mexico and California, also known as 'Brickellia Grandiflora herb' Prodigiosa. These plants/shrubs were used for the treatment of diarrhea, diabetes and stomach pain by the Mexican as a tea. Study carried out on Prodigiosa reveals that the plant is an antioxidant, produces chemical compounds that help secrete stimulation of the pancreatic gland and decreases or reduces the amount of blood sugar, helps absorb fat in the gallbladder, and also increases the health of the digestive tract of the stomach.

4. The root of a plant called Burdock that can be found all over the globe is Burdock root. Virtually all is essential about Burdock as its root is used as food and medicine and it uses leaves and seeds for medicinal purposes. Many people claim the oral intake of Burdock helps improve urinary flow, remove germs, purify blood, avoid and cure cancer, joint discomfort, colds, diabetes, anorexia, fever, bladder diseases, syphilis, gastrointestinal and intestinal complaints. This plant does not stop there, as it also helps to cure skin disorders such as acne and psoriasis and to avoid them. Burdock also helps to increase sex drive (libido), reduce high blood pressure and cleanse the lymphatic system and liver.

5. "Dandelion is a flowering plant that is a European native, also known as "Taraxacum officinale. In the warm climates of the Northern Hemisphere, it is usually found. For decades, these flowering plants have been used to treat swelling (inflammation) of the pancreas, tumors, tonsils (tonsillitis), arthritis, bladder or urethra, intestinal or hepatic disorders. Analysis has shown that because of the vitamins (A, B, C, E and K), minerals (iron, potassium, magnesium and calcium) and other compounds (polyphenols, chicory and chlorogenic acid) found in Dandelion, it has the ability to detoxify gallbladder, kidney and blood purification. It also dissolves kidney stones, treats diabetes and avoids liver and urinary disease relief and avoidance. It also provides chemicals that can improve the development of urine, which helps disinfect the urinary tract and prevents the creation of crystals in the urine.

6. Elderberry, or Sambucus nigra, is sometimes referred to as European elderberry or black elder. It is a flowering plant belonging to the genus Adoxaceae and is endemic to Europe. In Europe and many other parts of the world, these flowering plants are common. As long as 9 meters, this plant can grow. It is 30 foot tall and has lots of clusters known as elderflowers (white or cream-colored flowers). Elderberry leaves have

been used for the management of pain for several years. Swelling, inflammation, and stimulating the production of urine and causing sweat. Since it has also been used as a laxative, diuretic and to cause vomiting, the bark is not left behind.

7. Guaco is a climbing vine, also known by other names as "Guace or Vedolin or Cepu or Bejuco de finca or Liane Francois or Cipo caatinga." With different minerals and compounds, this climbing plant is abundant. It comes from the Asteraceae family and from the cordifolia genus. Its leaves are extremely nutritious and medicinal.

8. Mullein is a flavored drink plant also known as 'Aaron's rod, Candlewick, American mullein, Adam's flannel, Denseflower mullein, Candleflower, European or orange mullein, etc For centuries before now, this flavorful drink plant has been used for the treatment of various diseases, including asthma, tuberculosis, pneumonia, chills fever, gastrointestinal bleeding, colds, chronic chronic coughs and others

Natural herbal tea

It is essential, according to Dr. Sebi, to sustain a "consistent use of natural botanical remedies" and cleanse and detoxify the body by doing so. Although it is a significant step in your path to better wellness to use herbs and natural cures, you must also try to make the right changes to your dietary habits by following the list of prescribed foods.

List & Use

We have shown that a diet focused on plants is important for a balanced diet. But we can't just include fruits and vegetables when we talk about plants, currently there is an amazing number of herbs with a strong alkaline influence as well. We need to know how important they can be to our health: they have a real curing effect that stops many diseases and reverses them. Herbal medicine is a very old procedure that consists of a set of plant-based medicinal techniques; contemporary official medicine is often aware of the remarkable properties of many plants and uses them with many traditional medicines. Simply by infusions, we can presume much of their macronutrients in a perfectly normal manner, but we can't ignore them in our alkaline diet. I would like to note a very well-known plant: the chamomile. Many people use it to relax or sleep, but very few people know its major alkaline effect: your body raises acid production while you're nervous or concerned, so chamomile tea helps your body regulate its pH value thanks to its calming effect. In addition, chamomile battles arachidonic acid and a significant anti-inflammatory effect is the result. Alfalfa, also known as Lucerne, is a less well-known herb with an extremely high nutrient content. Its name means "Father of All Foods" and it literally includes a wide range of vitamins, minerals, proteins and essential amino acids. It helps you to reset your metabolism, beyond its alkalizing influence, and keep away from various common diseases. More precisely, it can:

- Lower level of cholesterol

- Improve the functionality of the immune system

- Purify your blood

- Promote digestion

- Remove allergies

- Alleviate all forms of arthritis

- Relieving migraines and headaches

You can drink alfalfa tea everyday and if you like, blend it with another flavored tea, as alfalfa is very mild in taste. Or in capsule shape, you might take this plant. Know that this herb can never be missed, whatever you decide, it is one of the best secrets of an incredible safe life. Another alkaline plant you can eat as tea or even as a salad is Dandelion. It facilitates weight loss and contains strong antioxidants, and is an important help against kidney stones. For this cause, I recommend that you consume this herb as a fresh vegetable, cooking delicious salads with other vegetables: Dandelion is very high in vitamin C and folic acid that are susceptible to heat. Of course, Dandelion is very inexpensive, you can harvest it quickly in the fields or grow it in your greenhouse, so you should seriously consider adding this herb to your safe daily diet. The one based on red clover is a specific and almost unknown medicinal herb tea. It includes isoflavones, natural phytoestrogens used to combat cancer, indigestion, asthma and bronchitis, with high antioxidant effects. Red clover is particularly ideal for women as it improves the reproductive wellbeing of women and may decrease the risk of breast cancer. There are many herbs that are completely undervalued: people generally assume that our dishes are only meant to add flavor, but they add far more than that. I think of parsley, basil, cilantro, oregano, sage and thyme, for starters. Nobody understands that there is more vitamin C in parsley than in oranges! Likewise, it has a very high proportion of vitamin K and a lot of iron. Basil emits high levels of eugenol, a potent anti-inflammatory, into our bloodstream, while oregano is one of the strongest suppliers of free-radical warfare. Lime, sarsaparilla, verbena, sage, and laurel can be among the other alkaline herbs that we may use to make excellent infusions. Laurel is a valid partner for respiratory ailments such as pneumonia, bronchitis, cough, and pharyngitis. Moreover, it has beneficial effects on the treatment of arteriosclerosis and artery disorders. You should also consider purchasing essential oil with antibacterial and anti-tussive properties.

How to track a diet

<u>Rules to Follow</u>

1. You need to strictly stick to his guidelines, which are present on his website, to obey Dr. Sebi's diet. Here is a list of his instructions below:

2. Do not eat or drink any food or ingredient not specified in the diet's approved list. It is not recommended when following a diet and can never be eaten.

3. Per day you have to drink almost one gallon (or more than three liters of water. A drink of spring water is advised.

4. One hour before taking your medications, you must take Dr. Sebi's mixtures or drugs.

5. Without any worry, you may take together any of Dr. Sebi's mixtures/products.

6. You need to strictly follow the dietary recommendations and take the mixtures/products of Dr. Sebi daily punctually.

7. You are not permitted to eat any food or hybrid items dependent on livestock.

8. Alcohol or other forms of milk product you are not supposed to eat.

9. You are not permitted to ingest wheat as mentioned in the nutritional guide, only natural growing grains.

10. In multiple health food markets, the grains alluded to in the dietary guide can be available in various ways, such as pasta and bread. They can be eaten by you.

11. Do not use fruits from cans; for eating, seedless fruits are also not recommended.

12. To reheat your meals, you are not allowed to use a microwave.

How the Body Prepares

It should be clear that it is a low-calorie diet that is limiting. Many individuals agree that it should not be used as a normal way to reduce weight for this cause, as it places so much tension on a new dieter's body. Weight reduction can be observed when it is low in calories and an active diet, so the person has to decide whether they are capable of handling a low caloric diet. Being too optimistic with this diet could become deadly, so be cautious if you want to try the diet!

Throughout one's entire life, this diet has been recommended to be adopted, which might not be practical with a novice dieter. For any diet, the odds are that the weight loss and benefits you see will be reversed if you start cutting food heavily and soon return to your old habit of eating unhealthy meals. This is also a possibility on this diet. Set realistic goals before starting and do not go too strongly. Second, let the body get used to it and then start achieving more aggressive targets.

Meal Plan

It can be overwhelming to start dieting, but here is a list of meal ideas from which you can copy. Follow it for the first few days so that you get used to the diet.

Breakfast

1. Agave Syrup Banana Pancakes (more than one is recommended).

2. A smoothie of strawberries and bananas with hemp seeds and water added.

3. Cooked coconut milk (pure) quinoa with agave syrup for sweetness (also add a fruit of your choice).

lunch

1. A salad with spinach, tomatoes, carrots, avocados, chickpeas, olive oil and herbal tea.

2. A spelt-flour pizza, Brazil nut cheese served with assorted veggies such as onions, etc.

3. A spelt pasta with assorted ingredients, and dressings of lime and olive oil.

Snack for the Evening

1. A cucumber-based smoothie, spinach, a few slices of ginger, and one or two apples.

2. Herbal tea, followed by your favorite fruit.

3. Spelt-and-teff flour blueberry muffins, coconut milk (pure), agave syrup, and blueberries.

Dinner

1. A wild rice stir-fry with your pick of vegetables.

2. A spelt flour bread burger; potatoes, onions, and vegetable kale; and a chickpea patty.

3. A dense vegetable soup made from mushrooms, zucchini, peppers, cloves, sea salt, onions and powdered seaweed.

Drink Water

Smoothies are a drink and you are ultimately serving your water consumption for the day by enjoying them. The diet of Dr. Sebi needs you to drink one gallon of water a day, but it can be challenging. A significant concern that may lead to anxiety is dehydration. You need to drink plenty of water to stop it, which the smoothie diet helps you with.

What you're not supposed to eat

- It is not permissible to eat foods not specified in the dietary guide. Some samples of foods of this nature are given below:

- Any canned food specified in the nutritional guide, be it fruit or vegetables,

- Fruits without seeds, like grapes

- Eggs are not allowed

- No type of dairy product is permitted,

- Fish is not authorized.

- Any type of poultry should not be consumed.

- Red meat is specifically forbidden.

- Soy goods, a supplement for beef, are also forbidden.

- No refined foods are approved,

- Food from restaurants and food delivered shall not be eaten

- There are no licenses for hybrid and fortified foods

- Wheat is not allowed

- The strict prohibition of white sugar

- Alcohol has been banned

- Yeast and its goods are not permitted

- Baking powder is not allowed,

They have left out some other diets and ingredients. To know what you have to eat, you just need to obey the dietary guide.

Prep for Alkaline Meal

The liver is one of the essential organs of the different body sections, as it has significant potential for body detoxification. Synthetics and other outside contaminants such as toxins and even defecation, pee, and sweat are expelled from the body via this body detoxification. These contaminants come from unhealthy foods that we eat, such as controlled and non-regular rich foods, alcoholic drinks that we ingest, cigarettes that we smoke, and even medications that we spend on anti-infection therapy and elective hormone drugs. These compounds are the ones that our bodies struggle every day to take away. The liver has to hold up before its capacity runs out, as there are many dangerous compounds within the body. When this is denied, the body can collect large quantities of toxins that cause numerous complications and diseases in the body. We should experience a detoxification diet and take considerable care of our liver to predict this and preserve outstanding fitness.

Either a three-day, seven-day, or twenty-one-day regimen can be completed with a liver detoxification schedule. This relies on a strong reliance on a diet of unprocessed and natural ground-grown ingredients, whole grains, and water treatment with ample water or liquid calculation. It will be possible to avoid nutrients high in fat or sugar, caffeine, liquor beverages, unnatural and human-made ingredients, narcotics, and low-quality foods, at any rate, seven days before the diet schedule.

One to Three Days: This is the time where you need to drink between ten to twelve glasses of water alongside often crushed lime juice to launch your fluid diet schedule. While owing to the weariness and slightness, it can also be difficult to perform this diet, moderate exercise can be included as a request to affix the procedure of flushing the toxins out of the body. In addition, you should stop getting in some form of milk or dairy product.

Four to six days: celery, apples, carrots, bananas, all of which could be combined into one juice, can be spent on new organic goods, vegetables and whole grains. Your option of leafy foods can be mixed into the juice. While healthier foods are eaten, there are also liquid options for about a few cups per day, such as natural teas. They should add cut and bubbled vegetables such as celery, carrots, broccoli, and spinach with respect to supper. Besides, you should also use soups that can be brought in at periodic intervals.

Seven days: The liquids are spent along with the leafy vegetables. By making them crude or steamed, they will all be able to be sorted. In addition, rosemary tea and dandelion choices can be consumed, which can be beneficial for this time.

As long as you stick with the plan, you will normally adjust the kinds of foods harvested from the soil that you can need. You will indulge in the traditional diet until the seventh day is a doe; eventually, though, following the detoxification diet, there is always a limit on liquor intake for about one full week. Once you experience temptation, disorder, and squeamishness, you must bring an end to the food. Quite definitely, this diet for detoxification will have an immense effect on the growth and development of a healthier lifestyle.

Detoxing your body with alternative therapies

In working out how to detox the body, traditional Chinese medicine (TCM) is a wonderful commodity and is primarily prescribed for the treatment of stomach-related issues, such as badly tempered inside syndrome; ceaseless skin disorders such as dermatitis; weariness and despair; hormonal painful disposition, such as PMS; endometriosis and low sperm count and barrenness (both male and female). With endless constraints, it can produce outcomes that Western approaches fail to support. It will make major changes to the health and prosperity of an individual at the moment when paired with a detox diet. Self-finding and management of illnesses are not recommended; however, you should portray the side effects to the expert behind the counter at any TCM focus points and get an effective remedy on the spot. TCM may be effective for helping people with abstinence from addictions to narcotics and liquor. Liquor creates uneven characters in the liver and nerve bladder, which identifies a combination of excessive moisture and water. Throughout the liver, several medicines are prepared, rendering it warm and blocked, so the blood of the liver becomes frail and inadequate. In order to help quiet the brain and sensory system, TCM calculations concentrate on clearing and supporting the liver and nerve bladder, while also treating the heart. Consolidating TCM is potentially the best thing you can do for your wellbeing by finding out how to detox your body yourself.

Chapter Three: Advantages of the Diet and Tips for Starting

The benefits of Dr. Sebi Alkaline

In maintaining the health of a person, the alkaline diet has a lot of benefits. Most of its benefits are provided by reducing unhealthy food consumption and eating more vegetables and fruits. Accompanying it with other healthy routines like exercise is to get the most out of any diet regimen. Starting an alkaline diet to improve your daily life is a great idea as we are drowning in bad health with our lazy lifestyle and fast foods. The following is a list of advantages that this diet can provide.

Loss of weight

This diet wasn't made with weight loss in mind, but you will see weight loss because it is extremely restrictive. Also one of the main reasons why this diet is effective in reducing weight is that it makes people stop eating highly caloric, oily, and sugary Western foods. Weight loss happens when you consume fewer or equal amounts of calories that can be burned. You can get your perfect body if you follow this diet that is low in sugar, fat, and processed foods. The causes of heart disease and also obesity are shown to be reduced by any diet whose main component is eating unprocessed plant-based foods. Except for some nuts and oils, the foods mentioned in this diet are low in calories. Even if you eat a large amount of them because of excessive hunger, your daily calorie intake will not be reduced by much. If you eat other types of food, weight gain and excessive eating will result. Only if you properly plan your servings and portion out ingredients can a constant state of weight loss be feasible. The diet does not provide this data, so planning your meals will depend on your management abilities.

Increases kidney function

The health of the kidneys is mostly affected by acidic diets and the layers within the organ system are damaged. The pH of the urine mustn't be acidic to promote kidney health. We can reach this pH at which our kidneys stay safe and healthy by consuming a lot of alkaline food and removing acidic foods from our daily routine. Alkaline diets have little effect on blood pH, but they may have a substantial influence on urine. Along with this diet, drinking a lot of water can improve the kidneys even more. If you have any chronic kidney disease, then you should know that you are not the target of this diet. After consulting with your doctor first you can follow the diet.

Reduces cancer risk

There are almost no important studies showing that an alkaline diet leads to reduced cancer cases. There have been lessons, however that show that if a person were to eat less meat and increase their intake of fresh fruits and vegetables, then that person is at a lower risk of cancer. Another study also showed that having more vitamins in your diet, like vitamin C, can prevent cancer. In general, eating more fruits and vegetables and eating less fatty and sugary foods leads to a decrease in cancer development.

Reduces heart disease risk

Heart disease is the world's major cause of death. It is primarily caused by eating lots of fat and oily foods, which leads to plaque development and artery blockage. The consumption of fats in this diet decreases significantly lowering the chances of developing heart disease. Growth hormones have also been shown to be related to decreased heart disease rates. An alkaline diet increases growth hormone levels, so it also decreases heart disease in turn.

Lowers the risk of degradation of muscles

We tend to increase muscle loss when we grow old or cease using our muscles. A study conducted in 2013, however, showed that individuals who follow an alkaline diet could reduce muscle degradation. The diet is low in red meat, so there is a risk that muscle mass and strength will decline.

Individuals eat more fruit and vegetables

People now lean towards fast and delicious treats and forget to eat fresh produce. Following this diet will lead to people consuming vegetables and fruits for their daily needs. We take in all their benefits and nutrition with the rise in their intake as well.

Increases health in the intestines

There is a list of nuts and seeds that you can eat on this diet with the addition of whole grains. It helps increase the intake of fiber, which improves the health of the small and large intestines. It helps to manage regular bowel movements, which lowers the risk of many diseases developing.

Reduces the damaging effects of processed foods

Increased sugar intake and fat content have been associated with processed foods. They also contain lots of calories, but their nutritional value is very low. If we strictly avoid processed foods, many additives and preservatives that have no purpose in our bodies are eliminated from our diets.

This aids the brain

Not only is the growth hormone associated with a better heart condition, but it also helps to manage the health of the mind. It is linked to an increase in cognition and memory. Eating a healthy diet rich in fruits and vegetables results in improved functioning of the brain.

Back pain can be improved

Alkaline minerals are linked to the reduction of back pain, but it has yet to be determined whether alkaline foods provide the same results. There is a decent chance that there will be similar effects from the diet.

Decreases inflammation levels

A great reduction in oxidative stress and inflammation is shown by diets rich in fresh fruits and vegetables. This results in less discomfort and the development of fewer diseases in our bodies.

Tips for starting the Diet of Dr. Sebi

The dietary guide from Dr. Sebi is very stringent, so before beginning this diet, one has to be mentally and emotionally prepared. It seems difficult to execute, but you will find yourself set for the trip until you have all the knowledge you need. Eating properly is a critical part of eating. The basic guidelines to follow, on a diet or not, are 3-5 meals a day, chewing properly, and not drinking water before your meals!

Digestion

To survive, humans require food. Fruits, fruits, fish, and other animals are the food we will find in nature. Digestion is a type of catabolism that lets us break down large molecules of food into small soluble molecules that will be ingested into the bloodstream and then into the cells, tissues and organs via the small intestines. With chewing, the digestive tract begins. The interaction of food with saliva begins digestion and creates the optimal pH conditions. The food is passed to the intestine, where it is converted into smaller molecules with the assistance of gastric acids and enzymes. The resultant substance reaches the duodenum within a few hours, where it begins to be digested with the help of pancreatic digestive enzymes and bile juice from the liver. The nutrients are ingested into the blood until digestion is over. Therefore, proteins are turned into amino acids, glucose into sugars, and lipids into fatty acids.

Metabolism

In everybody, metabolism is a series of chemical reactions. It's inspiring us:

- Conversion of essential food nutrients into energy

- Proteins, nucleic acids, lipids, and carbohydrates transform foods into

- Elimination of nitrogen waste

Every person requires food to survive, to have the ability to survive, to counteract toxic forces, to revitalize cells and tissues, and to extract toxins from the body. For humans, seeking food has always been a problem. Just a vegetarian regimen was used by the first humans on earth. Over time, they continued to hunt and fish. When the fire was found, people started to alter their diet, and now they had equipment to cultivate crops and raise livestock. People began consuming processed products such as sugar, flour, and other condensed foods in the 19th century. People began to use hybrid and genetically engineered crops in the 20th century due to selective farming and breeding of mutants.

Why is food so critical?

To receive the lipids, fats, vitamins, minerals, and carbohydrates that our body uses to synthesize into nutrients every day, we need food. We will acquire the necessary enzymes, amino acids, and other nutrients important for the functioning of our body with the aid of digestion. They'll keep us safe and resilient. We make the most of nutrients with the help of metabolism. In short, the sooner the tiny molecules are synthesized by our cells, muscles, and organs, the better our body remains in place. BAT (brown adipose tissue) would not have any time to form.

Mindset

Perhaps the best option for our diet is vegetables. Dr. Sebi probably thought so. He was in my humble view, absolutely right. Just us can help with natural foods. Additives, salt, sugar, and food preservatives are full of refined foods that are not entirely nutritious and are perhaps a major part of the high incidence of obesity and other health issues in the US. Of the world as a whole.

One may say: natural food depends on it! Yeah, Dr. Sebi Diet's dietary guide is stringent, certain products are not so easy to find in any store, but you will come to know that it is not that hard with a bit of patience. As in something worth fighting for, attitude is key!

You need to remember the weakness is a necessity when you try to lose weight, and challenges can still spring up when least anticipated. Try to reflect on your target and not on how constrained your food selections are. A big step ahead is getting mentally ready. It is not simple to change your eating habits. Regular patterns are deeply rooted in our subconscious, but we need to take the initiative to change them. Start with small steps and try to tell yourself that this is the correct way to accomplish your aspirations, loss of weight, and good wellbeing. Get your family and friends' encouragement, surround yourself with good people and move on step-by-step. Small improvements every day will lead to healthier eating habits for a lifetime.

Take more water

We all understand how liquids are important to our body's proper functioning. Depending on body size and age, the body includes from 55 percent to 78 percent water. For a month, we can survive without food, but we don't last longer than a couple of days without water. In addition to this fundamental position in life, we still use water to cleanse our bodies. It plays an essential role in sustaining a balanced brain, ensuring the proper functioning of the body, and removing toxins from the body. It is important to stay well hydrated. In reality, Dr. Sebi's supplements contain herbs that stimulate urination to remove contaminants, so you need to consume more water in order to replenish the eliminated water. He recommends that up to one gallon of water a day be drunk. In his view, because it's normally alkaline, spring water is the perfect option. High chloride levels and other toxins may be present in tap water.

Start reading labels for food

Knowing what we consume is a must for any lifestyle that we may adopt. In order for the trip to get tricky, we would have to deny ourselves of desired foods or beverages. Starting to read labels will make us realize that there is no need for junk food. Letting go of any normal meals or snacks that do not contain our required nutrients would become simpler. Knowing what you eat and drink will make you sure that you are making the best food decisions. Changing eating habits is going to come easily. The nice news is that you will be fully conscious of what you did wrong, what you ate, and shouldn't have in the event of a relapse (it's natural to experience it at some point!). It may sound dumb, but it's a chance to change your eating habits for good!

Whole foods

Of course, fresh fruits or vegetables, something you want from the nutritious guide of Dr. Sebi, is easy to prepare, mostly because most of them are better eaten raw. The concept is to resist canned or refined foods and slowly incorporate whole foods into our diet. Cooking your recipes will make you understand the value of the diet better. You will get great pleasure from preparing new recipes sometimes. Cooking your meals will make it easier for you to regain charge of the food you consume so that when seeking new approaches to your favorite dishes, you recover your wellbeing. The accepted ingredients in the nutrition guide from Dr. Sebi could bring spice to your life.

Snacks

Old practices are dying hard! Meat is the brain's security blanket. Our brain gives out signs of risk while on a diet, so we have to feed in those times. It is not always a bad thing to have snacks. It would work just fine if we have at least 6-7 fruit or vegetable snacks a day. One should eat an avocado, some olives, dried fruits, or cherry tomatoes instead of opting for a bag of chips. Our brain is happy, our body doesn't feel hunger anymore, and we remain lean and fit.

Old practices are dying hard! Meat is the brain's security blanket. Our brain gives out signs of risk while on a diet, so we have to feed in those times. It is not always a bad thing to have snacks. It would work just fine if we have at least 6-7 fruit or vegetable snacks a day. One should eat an avocado, some olives, dried fruits, or cherry tomatoes instead of opting for a bag of chips. Our brain is happy, our body doesn't feel hunger anymore, and we remain lean and fit.

Overall gain from Dr. Sebi diet

The Diet of Dr. Sebi is not yet another fad. Apart from weight reduction, it has many advantages. Let's find out how it can totally transform our lives to pursue this vegan, alkaline-based approach to food.

Weight

For most of us, weight loss is the big priority. Even if Dr. Sebi has not formulated this weight loss diet, we know that by following his rules, we will lose weight. The diet is focused on the intake of fruits and vegetables, which are rich in vitamins, nutrients, fiber, and other compounds associated with decreased inflammation, oxidative stress, and many diseases. A research has found that there was a reduced risk of cancer and heart disease among people who ate seven or more servings of fruits and vegetables a day. In comparison to the Western diet, this diet is focused on values that prohibit us from refined foods, dense fats, sugar, salt, and other unhealthy ingredients.

Detox

The Dr. Sebi Diet is also ideal for extracting the body from toxins and refined elements. Our body needs nourishment, and in nature we find all the food we need. But it is toxic to certain components of the foods we consume. Some become toxic to our bodies after they are processed. The consumption of beef, certain vegetables, dairy products, processed foods and other products results in the release of certain unhealthy components. These are a shortcut to serious conditions only. Dr. Sebi Diet's aim is to remove toxins that are bound to raise the risk of contracting these diseases. It will also assist us in enhancing our fitness, stamina, and strength. To repair any disruption or imbalances, intra-cellular washing is important to cleanse the body's processes at a cellular level. Imbalances primarily apply to dietary deficiency and disruption to your normal biochemical structure because of the deposition of excess toxins, enzymes, calcification, and mucus in the structures of the body.

Good eating habits

He has to face restrictions, straining physical workouts, and most notably, struggling with fresh food habits while one is on a diet. That's the hardest part—getting used to something different, something we've got to do. It can get tricky when someone orders you to do or not to do that! I mean, trust me. The optimistic point is that after just a few days, your body can get used to the new food regime. About why? We are vegetarians, even though that's what nobody tells you. Mother Nature has a way of supplying us with all that we need. Plants, plants, and humans are taken care of by her. It portrays, for Amerindians, the goddess of fertility who presides over planting and harvesting. If it was not made by god, don't take it! It is not easy to change your eating habits regardless, but you can find that if you obey some basic rules for some days, it is very easy. It would go automatically from there on!

Lower risk of chronic diseases

A reduced risk of cancer, elevated blood pressure, heart attacks, and type 2 diabetes is a possible advantage of this lifestyle. About why? Much of this is because of fresh diets that do not contain unhealthy nutrients.

Chapter four: Some disease and Dr Sebi herbal cure

With the Dr. Sebi's diet, there are couple of illnesses that look impossible to cure but can be treated when this diet is pplied properly and correctly to your daily lives. Some of these illnesses are:

Hypertension/ High blood pressure

Hypertension is a long-term clinical problem in which there is a constant rise in blood pressure. For strokes, heart disease, vision loss, and even dementia, it is a major risk factor. We have to stay away from meat and alcohol for the procedure, not drink too much tea, and consume fruits and vegetables authorized by Dr. Sebi. Olives, wild rice, cabbage, cucumbers, bell peppers, kale, squash, valerian, and chickpeas are the vegetables to purchase. For our diet, dried fruits are the perfect option.

Diabetes Type-2

Type 2 diabetes is a chronic condition that arises due to obesity, especially in individuals over the age of 40. It is characterized by insulin deficiency, which is a vital factor in digestion. We ought to keep away from fried foods, sugar teas, potatoes, and lentils to treat diabetes. Kale, cucumber, cabbage, cherry and plum tomatoes, chickpeas, bell peppers, squash, mushrooms, dandelion, and onions are the veggies to eat. Fruits such as red raspberry, plums, apples, and seeded key limes are what we can consume. Sour soups are strongly recommended for the treatment of type-2 diabetes.

Adiposity

Obesity is a chronic disorder in which cumulative extra body fat contributes to numerous disorders, such as type 2 diabetes, coronary problems, obstructive sleep apnea, osteoarthritis, depression, and even some cancer forms. Poor dietary habits, inactive lifestyle, biology, bowel flora, mental disorders, and social determinants are responsible for this. Eating fruits and vegetables, staying away from meat and alcohol, and consuming lots of liquids are the perfect remedies for obesity.

Ulcer of stress

An ulcer is a discontinuity in the membrane of the body that hinders the normal operation of the organ that is affected. The most prevalent form of ulcer encountered in all countries is stress ulcer. It primarily affects the stomach and can contribute to ulcerative perigastritis, massive bleeding, and stenosis. Dr. Sebi's remedy involves eating vegetables for their calming influence, such as tomatoes and squash, ripe fruits (apples, peaches, raisins), sour soups, and lots of herbal teas, especially fennel and chamomile.

Constipation

Constipation is a condition that affects our well-being deeply. Other risks, such as hemorrhoids and anal fissure, can arise from abdominal discomfort, bloating, and infrequent bowel movements. The remedy for Dr. Sebi consists of consuming fruits (primarily apples, peaches, plums, figs), vegetables (squash, kale, and chickpeas), basil, nuts, and plenty of herbal teas, especially fennel, dandelion, and chamomile.

Arteriosclerosis

Atherosclerosis is a condition that narrows the arteries and can lead to strokes, coronary heart disease, and complications with the kidneys. Alcohol intake and smoking are prohibited. Coffee should be minimal, but a valid boost is lettuce tea. We can eat wild rice, bananas, and vegetables, in addition to physical activity.

STDs and herpes

Herpes and all STDs are bacterial pathogens that the immune system is not able to overcome. Stable sex is the only form of prevention. Herbal teas such as burdock and dandelion, consuming a number of dates, and lettuce are part of Dr. Sebi's remedy.

Gout

Gout is inflammatory arthritis due to low uric acid levels in the blood, marked by frequent extreme pain, red hot, and swollen joints. It may contribute to kidney disease. We can mix fiber with uric acid in the digestive tract in this situation, so that it no longer produces deposits of crystals. To reduce gout, the most effective way is to lose weight, take plenty of supplements, and avoid alcohol. Dietary supplements do not have any effect on gout, according to experts, but Dr. Sebi recommends us to drink burdock, dandelion and elderberry teas. Consuming alkaline fruits and vegetables also tends to decrease the levels of uric acid.

GERD (disease of gastroesophageal reflux)

GERD is a long-term condition in which the substance of the intestine rises in the esophagus. Insufficient closing of the esophageal sphincter is the leading cause, but there is also obesity, obstructive sleep apnea, and gallstones involved. We need to improve our habits, eat better, start working out, avoid smoking, and most importantly let go of acidic foods. That's why the dietary guide from Dr. Sebi would give us a hand to resolve this ailment.

Asthma

Owing to excess deposition of mucus, environmental and genetic factors, asthma is a persistent inflammation of the longings. This is very difficult to stop, but easier to treat. Vitamins, amino acids, respiratory maneuvers, and breathing strategies are used in herbal medicine to ensure the proper operation of the lungs. Using fennel, anise, chamomile teas, and alkaline fruits and vegetables, Dr. Sebi tells us.

Top 10 foods that seem safe, but you need to avoid

Fruit juice

Many people use a glass of orange juice to start their day. Yeah, they oughtn't. It takes four oranges for a single glass of juice to be made. While juice is a nutritious beverage, all the fiber from the fruit has sadly been discarded. Besides, there is just as much sugar in fruit juice as in soft drinks. Eating an orange, not consuming a bottle of orange juice, would be a great way to start a day. That way, you will get all the vitamins, including the fiber, and it would be minimal to cope with the amount of fructose the liver needs to deal with.

Farmed salmon (Atlantic salmon)

Since it's rich in omega-3 fatty acids, most people eat salmon. Farmed salmon available today, though, have slightly lower levels of these good fats than the salmon we were only able to afford five years ago. The most plausible cause for this is that much less healthy food is now being fed to salmon. Besides in farmed salmon, dioxin levels are ten times higher than in wild salmon. This is bad news because cancer, organ injury, and dysfunction of the immune system are related to this compound.

Artificial sweetening agents

In certain sugar-free products, chemical sweeteners are included and gums, baked goods, jams, etc are chewed. Sugar substitutes, such as sorbitol, xylitol, mannitol, erythritol, maltitol, lactitol and isomalt, are all focused on them. While they are sold as natural, these artificial sweeteners are actually highly refined and are mostly made from GMO ingredients. Long-term use of artificial sweeteners can create a gut flora imbalance and lead to diabetes, gastrointestinal issues, weight gain, etc. On top of that, farmed salmon are fed with illegal pesticides on a daily basis. To make matters even worse, manufacturing and exporting genetically modified salmon without having to mark it as such has recently become legal.

Shrimp

A certain food additive that is used to enhance the color of shrimp is found in farmed shrimps. This additive has estrogen-like effects that can alter men's sperm count and increase women's risk of breast cancer. In addition, ponds, where shrimps are raised, are also handled with neurotoxic pesticides that are known to cause certain neurological disorders, signs of attention loss, memory failure, etc.

Milk that is fat-free and low-fat

It lacks a great deal of its nutrients as raw milk is pasteurized. Long-life milk is especially dangerous because at temperatures of around 1000 degrees Centigrade, it must first be dry, after which water is added to it. Needless to mention, no enzymes will withstand these high temperatures or any other nutrients. People typically prefer dairy products that are low-fat or fat-free so they don't want to add weight. What they don't know, though is that carbohydrates or sugar are added as fat is eliminated. This is done to add flavor to milk, otherwise it will taste like water. So, fat-free and low-fat milk has added sugar, which puts you at risk for developing diabetes or heart disease if you drink a lot of milk.

Coffee with flavors added

There are a range of health benefits to black coffee and it will also shield you from some liver disorders. However, once it has been applied to butter, whipped cream or condensed milk, it becomes a rather dangerous cocktail. When you add non-dairy liquid creamers dependent on corn syrup, it gets even more unhealthy. The healthiest choice is black coffee, and while these ingredients boost coffee flavor, they can lead to elevated liver fat and some gastrointestinal issues.

Seitan

We generally see seitan as a safe alternative to protein from beef. It is actually wheat gluten, though. This suggests that you may experience signs of gluten intolerance even if you are not allergic to gluten, but you also eat seitan. Besides, seitan, over 500 milligrams per 100 grams, contains a lot of sodium.

Canned green beans

For whatever excuse, some of the most toxic canned foods that exist are U.S.-grown canned green beans. Any of the most toxic chemicals are treated with this diet and consuming just one serving a day places you at risk of getting cancer and having other health issues. In addition, all containers are packed with Bisphenol A-containing products. This is a synthetic estrogen that may cause issues with pregnancy for both men and women. This is one of the ingredients you must stop at all times, whether you can find fresh or frozen green beans.

Diet soda

The key explanation that diet soda can be stopped is that it's made of chemical sweeteners. This is worse for your body than ordinary candy, for a variety of reasons. So you are at a greater risk of contracting both cancer and diabetes if you drink diet soda daily.

Non-organic strawberries

There are so many contaminants from pesticides and fertilizers in some fruits and vegetables that they are potentially harmful to consume. Strawberries are one of them. In addition to pesticides, the soil that grows non-organic strawberries is also treated with poisonous gases. These were designed for chemical weapons originally, but are now used in agriculture. In other words, keep away from them if you can't afford organic strawberries.

Approved Foods

We have seen how we can be improved by this diet. To get the best results, let's see what foods we can use. This diet's meal schedule is a very strict one. You should skip what is not on the list as much as possible

The Vegetables

Vegetables are sections of plants eaten as food by humans. They are mainly low in fat and starch, but high in fiber, vitamins and minerals. You would be encouraged by every nutritionist to eat at least five servings of vegetables a day. Vegetables provide a significant influence on the equilibrium between acidic and alkaline.

For the Dr. Sebi Diet, the vegetables are:

Asparagus

Asparagus is an ancient plant that is poor in calories and sodium but high in vitamins, dietary fibre, folic acid, potassium, and chromium, a mineral that governs insulin's ability to bring glucose from the bloodstream to the cells. Water makes up 93% of its composition; it is also used for diuretic properties as well. In salads, stir-fried, baked, or in soups, it can be eaten raw. It lacks much of its nutritional properties in soups. For any food that is boiling or over steamed, this law holds. Raw food, as Dr. Sebi claims, is the safest dietary option. The same law is applied by other nutritionists to their diets.

Amaranth

Amaranth may either be used as a vegetable leaf or as a crop. For our diet, we're going to use both! It is abundant in proteins, dietary fiber, minerals, and carbohydrates. It is low in fat and has no gluten. The easiest way to eat it is stir-fried, steamed, or raw. For biscuits, cereals, bread, crackers, and other baked goods, grains may be eaten boiled or ground into flour.

Avocado

The avocado is of American origin and high in vitamins, fats, and carotenoids. As a supplement for beef, it is prevalent in every vegetarian diet only because it has a high fat content. Avocado is usually eaten fresh, but it is used for juices and soups as well.

Bell peppers

Some of the sweetest vegetables are bell peppers (red, orange, white, purple, or yellow). They are native to, but are now grown worldwide in Central America, Mexico, and northern South America. They are rich in liquids, vitamins, and carbohydrates (94 percent), and low in fat and protein. For green salads and sandwiches, eaten mainly fresh, they make an elegant and eye-catching sauce. Stir-fried, baked, and steamed, these delicious vegetables are also good ways to eat them.

Cucumbers

An ancient vegetable with a mildly bitter taste and a mild melon flavor. Cucumbers are rich in water (95%), vitamins, and kilocalories, but poor in nutrients that are important. For this diet, we have to eat it raw because pickled cucumbers contain acidic additives and sugar that we have to hold at bay.

Chickpeas aka Garbanzo beans

In sandwiches, soups, hummus (the main ingredient), and ground into rice, chickpeas are used. It is an ancient plant rich in protein, nutritional fibre, minerals, vitamins and essential amino acids. They are 60% water and are low in fat. In general, they are eaten boiled easily for 10 minutes and then simmered for a long time. It is used both deliciously and nutritiously in salads, soups, processed into flour, and as an ingredient for veggie burgers, much like amaranth grains.

Chayote

Chayote is an American-origin edible plant rich in vitamins and amino acids. It can be eaten raw, baked much like summer squash, or stir-fried in salads and salsas. Generally, we consume fruit, but shoots and leaves are also used for salads or stir-fries in certain countries. Due to its diuretic and anti-inflammatory properties, it is used in the Dr. Sebi Diet. To treat hypertension, remove kidney stones, and treat arteriosclerosis, tea made of Chayote leaves is used. For detoxifying our bodies, these are important properties.

Dandelion greens

Dandelion is native to North America and is used as food and medicine in Eurasia. It is rich in calcium and vitamins. 86 percent liquids, sugars, modest levels of protein and relatively low fat are contained. The whole plant is nutritious, but the leaves are the only ones we can use. They have a bitter flavor, but they make our green salads an excellent ingredient. The most popular part of all diets, primarily for weight loss, is in the Mediterranean region. It's high in calcium, so it's important for bone development and strength. Dandelion also improves the functioning of the liver, prevents it from ageing, and treats bleeding in the liver. It has been used in China, America and Europe in western medicine. For liver diseases, urinary disorders, diabetes, anemia, jaundice, and certain cancers, Dandelion is healthy. Dandelion powder is used to improve the production of urine and as a laxative. It is the ultimate toner for the skin, tonic for blood, and tonic for digestion. It includes alkaline chemicals that make it an outstanding anti-inflammatory agent. It is used by certain persons for lack of appetite, knee pain, bruises, stomach pressure, and gallstones.

Kale

The Mediterranean and Asian roots of kale or leaf cabbage have been grown for centuries for fruit. It is rich in sugars, vitamins, carotenoids, dietary minerals, and low in fat and proteins. It is made of 84% water and can be consumed raw, steamed, or stir-fried. Stir-frying or steaming so the amounts of glycosylate compounds that are potentially harmful to our wellbeing are minimized. For now, evidence has not yet shown that our health is affected by it. All we know so far is that kale, recommended by nutritionists or not, is used in every diet. Mediterranean diet, the diet of Sirtfood, and even the diet of Dr. Sebi. For sandwiches, veggie tacos, pasta and smoothies, kale is a delicious ingredient.

Lettuce

Originally farmed by ancient Egyptians, lettuce is a leaf vegetable used for fruit and medicine. Lettuce, which is usually consumed fresh, is a healthy source of vitamins, beta-carotene, folate, and iron. Typhoid, smallpox, rheumatism, nervousness, and cough have been used in medicine, but little scientific evidence has been identified to date.

Mexican squash

In soups, pickled, baked, grilled, spaghetti, pizzas, and even raw-in salads, sliced or shredded-Mexican squash is a vegetable used for cooking. It has a low kilocaloric content, but is rich in vitamins, potassium and folate.

Mushrooms (with Shiitake exception)

The mushroom is a fungus's fleshy fruiting body. They are high in water, sugars, and vitamins (92 percent), but low in proteins and fat. Edible mushrooms are used worldwide for their delicious taste in cuisine. Pay heed to mushrooms that are poisonous or hallucinogenic! They are used, even though there is no evidence of health effects, in traditional Chinese medicine.

Onions

Onions are vegetables used as food and as medicine, of ancient Asian origins. They are used to heal oral sores, sleep disturbances, ocular ailments, dysentery, and lumbago. It is one of the most well recognized natural antibiotics worldwide. They are around 89% liquids, rich in carbohydrates, and low in fiber, proteins, and fat in the diet.

Okra

Okra is an edible seed pod, high in carbohydrates, vitamins, dietary fibre, and poor in proteins and fat, of Asian or South African roots. We will use both the leaves and the seeds for our diet. It ends in slime when the seed pods are fried, and that paste contains soluble fiber. You should use an acid to "slime" it but it is better to eat it raw or used in salads since we want to preserve our body's alkaline condition. Okra is high in water (90%), sugars, folate, and vitamins, and low in protein and fat. We can eat the leaves and seeds as well.

Olives

The olive tree is an ancient tree, and the main component in Mediterranean cuisine is its fruits. We should use olives and olive oil in our diet, which is a must for any diet. Olives (75 percent) are an essential source of calories, vitamins and water, but they are poor in proteins and carbohydrates.

Purslane

Purslane, aka duckweed, is a vegetable that can be eaten raw, stir-fried, baked, or in soups and stews, of European and North African roots. It is rich in vitamins, high in water (93 percent), sugars, calcium and magnesium, but low in fat and proteins.

Squash

The squash has Central American origins, and because of their edible fruits and seeds, only five varieties are grown. Raw squash is water at 94 percent. It is a rich source of vitamins and food minerals, such as nutrients. It is low in fat and proteins. There are vitamins, saturated oils, and fatty acids in the grains. For cakes, puddings, cookies, salads, soups, bread, and the famous pumpkin pie, it is a flavorful ingredient. It's better to eat it raw, but it also fits with stir-fried or lightly steamed rice.

Sea vegetables, aka algae

(Kelp/Dulse/Nori/Wakame)Seaweeds are marine algae with up to 90% of the Earth's oxygen producing a crucial role. There are only certain animals that are edible. They can be used for cakes, drinks, dressings for salads, sauces and baked goods. They're fantastic dietetic ingredients. They are used in medicine because they keep certain DNA and RNA-enveloped viruses at bay. The pills made from seaweed extract have the same effect as gastric banding-they stretch and make it feel full in the stomach.

Tomatoes (only Cherry & Plum)

Any of the tastier plants on Earth, with South American origins, are tomatoes. Tomatoes can also be very acidic, even though they have the sweetest flavor, so Dr. Sebi recommended only using cherry and plum varieties for our diet. We're not going to be eating more acidic foods than we need in this manner. They are a moderate source of vitamins, but are poor in fat, proteins and carbohydrates. They are 95% water.

Tomatillo

The tomatillo is identical to peppers, aka the Mexican husk tomato. It has the same water content (95%); it's rich in vitamins and low in fat and protein. In many dishes, they are eaten raw or fried, particularly in salsa verde, but also in soups, salads, stir-fries, and desserts. They can also be dried to maximize the fruit's sweetness. Raw, yellow, or green tomatillo transforms into a varied green salad dressing that is delicious and eye-catching.

Wild arugula

Arugula, aka missile, has European and Asian roots and is from the mustard tribe. It grows wildly in regions of temperate climates. It is rich in vitamins, carotenoids, polyphenols, and ascorbic acid, but poor in protein and fat. Arugula is 92% water. For green salads, it has a spicy, pungent taste that makes it the best choice. Consume it raw or stir-fried only; if not all its properties and distinguished flavor would be lost. For pizzas, pasta dishes, or soups, it is a perfect ingredient. It is used in medicine to cure gastroenteritis and control the passage of the intestine.

Zucchini

The zucchini, first grown in the 19th century, is the Italian variety of squash. It is rich in potassium, folate, and vitamins, but low in fat and proteins. Fresh (sliced or shredded), steamed, roasted, stir-fried, and baked in various dishes may be served. It's a delicious compliment to green salads. It can be pickled as well but because pickles contain acid additives, that's not ideal for our diet.

Approved Fruits

Fruits are Mother Nature's blessing as well. They are a substantial source of human food. They also contain fibres, water, and vitamins, except for their sweet taste (they are moderately high in sugar). For stomach secretions and hunger, they are also a perfect stimulus. For the draining of the liver and digestive tract, fruits are also useful, providing a major effect on the peristalsis to evacuate the intestinal material and stop constipation.

For the Dr. Sebi Diet, the fruits are:

Apples

Apples are fruits of ancient Asian origin that are now grown worldwide. It is rich in water (86%), a modest source of dietary fiber, carbohydrates, and poor in micronutrients, fat, and protein content. It is used for cakes, juices or items that have been cooked.

Bananas

Bananas, introduced in the 16th century to the Americas, are one of the sweetest fruits on Earth, of Austronesian origins. The positive thing is that they are open during the year. Water (75%), potassium, vitamins, and carbohydrates, a modest source of dietary fiber, and poor in protein and fat, are quite high. It is usually eaten raw, but it is often used in flour for smoothies, cakes, or roasted, deep-fried, baked, steamed, or ground.

Cherries

In Europe, Asia and North Africa, cherries have been eaten since prehistoric times. In the 15th century, they were brought to the Americas. A moderate source of carbohydrates, vitamins, and dietary fiber, sweet cherries are 82 percent water, and are low in protein and fat. Instead, sour cherries contain more beta-carotene and more vitamins. For drinks and sweets, they may also be used.

Cantaloupe

Cantaloupe, also known as sweet melon, has Asian roots, and is now globally available. It is 90 percent water, high in vitamins, poor in calories, proteins and carbohydrates. They eat the fruit raw, in salads, or as a snack. Also the seeds are edible. Dried and baked softly, they make an ideal snack.

Cactus fruit

Cactus fruit, usually referred to as prickly pear, is found in different kinds in the Americas. It has 88 percent water, a modest source of protein and fat-lowing carbohydrates, dietary minerals and vitamins. It is used in the form of salads, soups, snacks, drinks, candy, and beverages. In medicine, it is used as a coagulant for open wounds and for the treatment of urinary and digestive tract inflammation. Analysis has shown that it helps prevent diabetes, metabolic syndrome, cardiovascular disease, obesity, and some cancers. There is an explanation, then for Dr. Sebi's decision to use this fruit. Cactus fruit intake has also been found to result in decreased body circumference and BMI (body mass index).

Currants

As for their edible berries, the currants are grown. Ribes and black currants are our diet's best options. They are of European and Asian descent and are 82% water, a rich source of carbohydrates, iron and vitamins, and poor in fat and protein. Their seeds are high in fatty acids that are unsaturated. They are used in medicine to cure renal disorders and for menstrual and menopausal issues.

Dates

Dates, brought to Mexico and California in 1765, had ancient Northern African origins. The perfect option for any diet, including ours, is Medjool dates. For different desserts and puddings, dates may be eaten raw or baked. Stir-fried, dehydrated, ground into rice, or as juice may be used. They are a moderate source of protein, fiber, potassium, manganese, selenium, and zinc and have a sugar content of 80%. Study on mice has shown that DNA damage is minimized by the aqueous extract of date seeds.

Figs

Figs are native to the Mediterranean region and Asia. Monosaccharide sugars and mixed phytochemicals such as flavonoids, rutin, and chlorogenic acid are found in the fruits. Dried fruits contain higher levels of polyphenols and sugar.

Mango

Mango is a juicy fruit native to South Asia that has now spread worldwide. It is a rich source of nutrients such as vitamins, folate, and others. It includes polyphenols and carotenoids. In pies and sauces, it can be consumed raw as a fruit, in juices and ice cream, pickled, or fried.

Oranges

Oranges, introduced into the Americas in the 15th century, are native to Asia and can be consumed fresh, processed for juice, oils, and marmalade. Vitamins, carotenoids, flavonoids, and various volatile organic compounds are rich in them.

Papayas

Papayas are native to Central America and can only be eaten raw whether they are peeled or fried. Even the black seeds are edible and taste spicy. They contain 88% water and are an essential source of vitamins, folate and carbohydrates, but they are poor in protein and fat. It has been used for treating malaria, relieving asthma, or as a purgative in herbal medicine. All those uses, according to Dr. Sebi, make it a perfect option for our diet.

Plums

Fruits linked to peaches and cherries are plums. With a wide number of animals, they have ancient European and Asian origins. A moderate source of vitamins and carbohydrates but poor in fat and proteins, they are 87 percent water. It functions just fine for the control of the intestinal tract in medicine used as a purgative.

Pears

Ever since ancient times, pears have been used. Their roots are Chinese and are used raw, frozen, or dried in juices. It is a moderate source of nutrients, minerals and dietary fibre, but it contains low amounts of proteins and fat. A pear is 84% water.

Peaches

Peaches are also native to China and were introduced in the 16th century to the Americas, and are perhaps the juiciest crop. They are 89% water, a moderate source of carbohydrates and vital nutrients, but they are poor in fat, protein, and calories. They are high in chlorogenic acid, rutin, and polyphenols.

Prunes

Prunes are plums which are fried. They are 31% water, high in sugars, nutritional nutrients and vitamins, but they are very poor in protein and fat.

seeded grapes

Grapes are delicious, juicy, Eastern-origin fruits that are grown for fruit or wine, jam juices, vinegar, and grape seed oil. A moderate source of carbohydrates, vitamins, and calories, grapes are 81 percent water, but poor in fat and proteins. There are good omega-3 fatty acids in the grape seeds and twice the polyphenol content in the grape skin. They are filled with vitamins and finely enriched nutrients. So we must use only seeded grapes for our diet. They are helpful for the wellbeing of the heart and brain and are beneficial for the skin.

Seeded key limes

For their special taste, key limes are prized. They are native to Southeast Asia, and has now expanded worldwide. Limes are 88% water, a rich source of vitamins, a modest source of carbohydrates and polyphenols, but they are very poor in proteins and fats. Seeds are more vitamin-rich and lower in acids. They can be eaten fresh as fruit or juices, or dried for exotic recipes, particularly desserts, as a flavor.

Seeded melons

Melons are juicy, soft, and fleshy fruits of a wide range of species and Central American origins. They are rich in vitamins and low in fat and proteins. They have a high natural sugar content.

Seeded raisins

The best ones for delicious treats are grapes or dried grapes. They are helpful for the wellbeing of the heart and brain and are beneficial for the skin.

Coconuts of soft jelly

Fruits grown in Jamaica are soft jelly coconuts; the edible component inside is generally called jelly. It is a large source of dietary fibre, but it is poor in proteins, calories, and carbohydrates. It can be used both for salads, snacks and drinks on its own and as an ingredient. It is used for digestive system control and detoxification of the internal organs

Sour (European or Asian markets) soups

Sour soups are used for their sour flavor in Eastern Europe and Asian cuisine. They contain mostly natural ingredients with a mildly acidic taste.

Tamarind

Tamarind has African roots and produces sweet and tangy pulp from pod-like fruits. It is an essential source of vitamins, starch, tartaric acid, and calcium. Some think the fruit to be too bitter, but for many savory recipes, it is included. It is used in medicine for its laxative properties and as a catapult for fever patients. Analysis has shown that it has antioxidant properties for the coagulation mechanism and antimicrobial reaction, and that it is effective in liver diseases.

Grain

Only whole grains are best, not processed ones, as described above. Carbohydrates, minerals, and dietary fiber are rich in them. In the type of pasta, cereal, flour or toast, you are required to eat grains.

The accepted grains are for the Dr. Sebi Diet:

Amaranth

The grains of amaranth are rich in dietary nutrients, have a modest intake of protein and carbohydrates, and are very low in fat.

Fonio

Fonio is a notable crop, mostly grown in countries of West Africa, known as 'hungry rice.' The grains are used for beer and fruit. They are highly nutritious, low in dietary fiber, and gluten-free.

Kamut (Khorasan wheat)

The Oriental type of wheat is Kamut. It has Oriental roots and a rich taste that is nutty. It is moderately nutritious, but poor in fat; it is a moderate source of protein, dietary fiber, vitamins and minerals. The other negative thing is that it includes gluten, meaning it's unacceptable for persons with gluten-related conditions.

Quinoa

Quinoa is part of a family of amaranths of South American origins. A modest source of protein, potassium, and low in calories, it is rich in carbohydrates, folate, and dietary minerals. Gluten-free is quinoa.

Rye

Rye is a grass cultivated for its grains, used for flour, bread, and alcoholic beverages, of ancient Eastern roots. It is high in proteins and calories, but poor in carbohydrates, dietary fibre, and vitamins. It is not poor in gluten, but it is unacceptable for those with gluten-related conditions. It is known for controlling blood sugar in medicine and raising cholesterol levels.

Spelt

The spelt is yet another form of wheat imported into the States only in the 19th century, an old grain in Europe. As a 'health food,' it has now found a new niche. It is a large source of protein, dietary fibre, starch, and vitamins. Sadly, it also includes gluten, meaning it's a concern for people with gluten-related conditions. For baked goods, it is commonly used as flour and is very easy to find in bakeries.

Teff

Another African grass, grown for its edible seeds, is Teff. Although low in fat, it is an essential source of carbohydrates, proteins, dietary fiber, and manganese. It is gluten-free and can be used in Ethiopian community as flour for bread, other baked goods, and alcoholic beverages.

Wild rice

In China and North America, wild rice is a semi-aquatic herb that has traditionally been consumed. It is a moderate source of dietary fiber, amino acids, and proteins, but is deficient in vitamins, iron, potassium, and fat. It doesn't contain gluten. It is possible to stew the grains or steam them.

Seeds and nuts

Nuts and seeds are crops that are energy-dense and nutrient-rich. For our diet, the nuts and seeds that are accepted are:

Brazil nuts

The Brazil nut is a South American tree that is responsible for the rise in HDL (good cholesterol), known for its high selenium content. It is also a rich source of proteins, dietary fibre, omega-6 fatty acids, vitamins and minerals.

Hemp seed

Hemp is one of Asia and Europe's first plants to be grown. In the 15th century, it was adopted into the Americas. It is possible to eat hemp seeds fresh, processed into dried powder, or as a liquid for drinks. In the US since 2000, hemp seeds have been used lawfully in food goods. They are rich in carbohydrates but low in calories, fats, dietary fiber, vitamins, iron, zinc, and fat. It is considered a good replacement for beef, milk, eggs, and soy when it comes to the protein content that hemp guarantees.

Raw sesame seeds

Sesame is one of the oldest recognized oilseed crops, famous for its rich and nutty taste, with Indian roots. It is one of the most commonly used spices in kitchens around the world. Carbohydrates, fat, vitamins, and dietary minerals are high in sesame seeds. In proteins, they are tiny. Sesame intake in medicine results in minor decreases in systolic and diastolic blood pressure, indicators of oxidative stress, and lipid peroxidation.

Raw sesame "Tahini" butter

Tahini is a condiment made from toasted or raw sesame seeds. As an organic food option, Raw Tahini is sold. It is a rich source of dietary nutrients, calcium, and proteins, mainly found in the Eastern, Mediterranean, and North African cuisines. In every vegetarian and vegan diet, and particularly in ours, when consumed raw, it makes a useful addition.

Walnuts

For decades, walnuts have been used in cooking all over the world. They are a common addition to savory meals, desserts, or for alcohol drinks in some nations, eaten raw or toasted. They've got a savory smell, which makes them an intriguing salad dressing. Fat, sugars, dietary minerals and vitamins are high among them. They are a modest source of dietary fiber and proteins. Non-conclusive evidence has shown that walnut intake decreases the risk of coronary heart disease. The thing that we know for sure is that brain food and very natural antibiotics are walnuts. Walnuts are used in herbal medicine to cure some heart problems, and even tumors, but there is little clinical evidence. Dr. Sebi believed that Candida cures and all parasites are destroyed by it. For safe digestion and bowel regularity, Walnut Hulls powder is used. It's still a good detoxifier, and it allows us to regulate the levels of blood sugar.

Oils

Edible oils are rich in alkaloids and proteins. They are used in food processing and in cooking for different reasons. The approved oils are for our diet:

Avocado oil

Avocado oil is an edible oil used in all manner of dishes or as cooking oil as an ingredient. It is not derived from seeds, but from the fruit's fleshy pulp. It is rich in insaturated fats, carotenoids, and vitamins. Naturally, it is poor in acid, making it a healthy option for Dr. Sebi's diet. We will use it to stir fried, barbecue, deep fry, and saute our meals.

(uncooked) coconut oil

Coconut oil is an edible oil extracted from mature coconut kernels or meat. It is rich in fatty acids, which is why we are urged to reduce intake slightly. Because of the high caloric properties of this oil, the FDA and other health organisations focus on the increased risk of cardiovascular problems and weight gain. In fact, clinical tests have shown that coconut oil intake contributes to higher LDL (bad cholesterol) levels, so it should not be perceived as a safe oil. As a cooking oil, only RBD (refined, bleached and deodorized) coconut oil can be used.

Grapeseed oil

Grapeseed oil is made of seeds that have been pressed. It can be used as a cooking oil, as a salad dressing, as a basis for herbal and spicy oil infusions, and in baked goods. It is comparatively high in fatty acids, polyphenols, and low in vitamins and saturated fats. Scientific evidence of health effects does not exist.

Hemp seed oil

Fat, sugars, dietary minerals and vitamins are high among them. They are a modest source of dietary fiber and proteins. Non-conclusive evidence has shown that walnut intake decreases the risk of coronary heart disease. The thing that we know for sure is that brain food and very natural antibiotics are walnuts. Walnuts are used in herbal medicine to cure some heart problems, and even tumors, but there is little clinical evidence. Dr. Sebi believed that Candida cures and all parasites are destroyed by it. For safe digestion and bowel regularity, Walnut Hulls powder is used. It's still a good detoxifier, and it allows us to regulate the levels of blood sugar.

(uncooked) olive oil

Olive oil is derived from pressed olives and is one of Mediterranean cuisine's main ingredients. It is used as cooking oil, but we just have to use it uncooked in our diet, so we make the most of its characteristics. For all kinds of dishes, it is the right complement to green salads and an additive. It is very high in fatty acids, very low in fiber and protein and of course, low in acidity. So far there is no empirical proof of its health effects.

Sesame oil

Sesame oil is an edible oil that, due to its nutty taste, can be used as cooking oil or as a spice for all kinds of dishes. Fatty acids, vitamins, and calories are extremely high in it. It is used in alternative medicines to get rid of fever. In order to attest to the effect on inflammation and atherosclerosis, experiments have been performed but without definitive findings.

Approved Herbs

Herbal teas

Herbs have been used as narcotics since ancient times, often for a good cause. They're working! They are plants with savory or aromatic properties which as a source of relief or for medicinal purposes, are used to flavor foods or as teas. Herbal teas include caffeine-a central nervous system (CNS) stimulant, astringent-acting tannins, and mineral salts. In addition to tea, you are free to drink as much water as you want. This encourages the separation from the body of unhealthy elements and increases the weight loss. Liquids ensure the function of the liver and most specifically, diuresis.

Mind, as soon as possible, to use distilled water! The authorised herbal teas are for the Dr. Sebi Diet:

Anise

Anise is a spice of Eastern origin, cultivated primarily because of its seeds. It is rich in protein and is therefore moderately high in dietary fiber and fatty acids. A regulator of digestion is known to be tea from whole or ground seeds, alone or mixed with other herbs. It also has diuretic effects that can be used to aid patients who suffer from insomnia or as a tranquilizer.

Burdock

Burdock is a native of Europe and Asia, comparable to an artichoke, noted for its sweet yet pungent taste. It is possible to consume the entire herb, but we will use tea from dried leaves. It is rich in fiber, potassium, and amino acids from the diet, but low in calories. It is used as a diuretic and a blood purifying agent in herbal medicine. It also reduces the level of cholesterol and stimulates the activity of the liver. As it destroys fungi and bacteria, burdock roots are used for acne, psoriasis, and carbuncles. And, it can be used as a skin diuretic and detoxifier.

Chamomile

Chamomile is an old plant that in most countries is growing wildly. Its flowers are rich in essential oils and polyphenols. It is used in herbal medicine for the prevention of insomnia. So far, clinical trials have shown no confirmation of its possible anti-anxiety properties. In digestive system disorders, stomach ulcers, and colic, its anti-inflammatory properties are effective. Chamomile tea has an anti-inflammatory effect and is a perfect antiseptic. It is also used to treat ADHD, fibromyalgia, hay fever, nervous asthma, and other sleep disturbances, as well as to relax the central nervous system.

Elderberry

The berries, leaves and flowers of the elderberry are grown. It is high in water (80%), sugars, vitamins, but poor in fat, proteins, and calories. Elderberry tea is used in medicine as a herbal supplement to cure colds, fever, and constipation. It is the number one enemy of mucus aggregation. It is also good for improving the immune system, which is why Dr Sebi believed that it could cure AIDS. The only other conditions that elderberries can cure are back and leg pain, nerve pain, and chronic fatigue syndrome.

Fennel

Fennel is an aromatic herb with a taste similar to anise, grown worldwide for its edible leaves and fruits. It is high in dietary fiber, carbohydrates, and vitamins, but is relatively low in protein and fat. The high content of volatile oils and phytochemicals such as rosmarinic acid and luteolin is the product of its fragrance. It can be used as a vegetable (from dried leaves or seeds), as a spice, and as an aromatic tea. It has been used since ancient times as a diuretic in herbal medicine.

Ginger

Ginger is an Asian-origin fragrant spice, bred for its aromatic origins. As a medicine, it can be used as a vegetable, juice, and alcoholic beverages. Ginger, a mild source of carbohydrates, vitamins, and dietary minerals, is 79 percent sugar, but poor in proteins and fat. Ginger herb tea is used for keeping chemotherapy or pregnancy-related nausea at bay. It is also used in osteoarthritis for its anti-inflammatory effects and for relieving pain. There is no direct proof of such consequences so far.

Red raspberry

A sweet, edible fruit, often cultivated for its leaves, is red raspberry, aka European raspberry. For its fruits, leaves and roots, the red raspberry is cultivated. It is a rich source of antioxidants, vitamins, potassium, iron and magnesium, and tea is used to destroy cancer cells in the stomach and colon. Any studies on mice found that intake of red raspberry stopped the development of kidney stones. It is also used as a skin-whitening agent in medicine. Women use it to relieve fatigue, leg cramps, and enhance sleep during breastfeeding because of its positive effect on the digestive system. It also has effects on the uterus and pelvic muscles, resulting in labour that is shorter and smoother.

Tilia

Tilia, also known as basswood, is an ancient tree famous both in Europe and North America for its flowers and blossoms, which are very popular in traditional medicine. Owing to the volatile oil that it contains, it has a very flavorful taste. It is used for its properties, both antioxidant and astringent. For colds, pneumonia, infections, fever, high blood pressure, and migraines, tea from the leaves and flowers is used. It is also used as a diuretic, antispasmodic, and sedative. Wood-based tea is used to cure digestive disorders, to protect the liver, and to treat gallbladder conditions and illnesses such as cellulitis or lower leg ulcers.

Spices

Spices are pieces of a herb that our foods are using for flavoring. In pharmacy, they are also used. They are poor in calories, sugar, protein and carbohydrates, but they are high in vitamins, minerals and micronutrients. They have antioxidant effects as well. The convenient aspect of including spices in a diet is that they are the intestinal secretions' primary "excitors." The spices we have to use are for our diet:

Achiote

Achiote is a South American tree used to colour meats, soaps, cosmetics, and medicinal products as a seasoning and a natural dye. Beta-carotene, essential oils, vitamins and fatty acids are high in it. It has been used for decades for its medicinal properties in herbal medicine.

Basil

Basil, of African and Asian roots, is a culinary plant. It has a distinct scent and taste that is sweet yet pungent. It is rich in essential oils and perhaps the world's most popular seasoning, used with all kinds of dishes and certain beverages. It has been used, much like achiote, in herbal medicine.

Bay leaf

Bay leaf is just another common spice used worldwide in cuisine, with different species and different flavors. It is moderately high in lauric acid and essential oils.

Cloves

In the Mediterranean, Asian, African, and Eastern cuisine, cloves are the flower buds of an Indonesian oak, used as a spice. It is rich in tannins, oleanolic acid, and essential oils. It also has certain bioactive compounds, making it a natural repellent for insects. The essential oil has been used as an analgesic or in aromatherapy in herbal medicine. But there is no clinical proof that except for alveolar osteitis, it acts as an analgesic for any discomfort. It also lacks definitive evidence from research on lowering fever or blood sugar levels. In particular, since it may cause side effects in patients with liver disease, immune system disorders, and food allergies, the FDA has not allowed its use for medical purposes.

Cayenne

A spice or herbal substitute, in its fresh nature or as a dried powder, is used for Cayenne peppers.

Dill

In all countries, dill is possibly one of the most common spices. It has Eurasian roots, with leaves and seeds grown for it. It is comparatively high, but poor in fat and protein, in carbohydrates, vitamins, and dietary minerals. It has been used in herbal medicine for its antibacterial properties.

Habanero

Habanero is yet another variety of South American-origin chili peppers. It is moderately rich in vitamins and carbohydrates, but poor in proteins and fat. It contains capsaicin, which is a compound found in dermal patches as an analgesic.

Oregano

Oregano, used as a seasoning for its flavorful fragrance, has Eurasian and Mediterranean roots. It is a key Italian cuisine ingredient. It has a high concentration of essential oils, carvacrol, and thymol.

Onion powder

Onions, now cultivated all over the world, are vegetables of Asian roots. A spice or herbal substitute, in its fresh nature or as a dried powder, is used for Cayenne peppers.

Sage

Sage is a herb of Mediterranean origin, now cultivated for its culinary and medicinal use worldwide. It is used in medicine as a pain killer and has therapeutic effects on the human brain.

Savory

Savory is a herb that is used in cooking and medicine of Mediterranean origins. It contains Carvacrol, a biochemical antibacterial agent. It has properties that are antiseptic, carminative, and digestive. For colic, gastroenteritis, cough, bronchial cough, sore throat, and inflammation, it is used as a remedy.

Thyme

Thyme is an ancient herb of European origin that has been used for centuries in cuisine and medicine. It is rich in essential oils, thymol in particular. It has been used in herbal medicine for its antiseptic properties.

Tarragon

Tarragon is a herb of Eurasian origin, now cultivated for medical and culinary uses worldwide. An antibacterial biochemical with possible anti-tumor effects, it is rich in phenylpropanoids, essential oils, and capillin.

Main Dr. Sebi herbs

Here is a list of the most herbs used by Dr. Sebi for natural healing, in addition to the herbal teas listed above.

Sarsaparilla root herb

Sarsaparilla, used as a basis for a soft drink and root beer, is a herb of Central American origin. It contains iron, beta-sitosterol, and saponins, which have anti-inflammatory effects that protect the liver. It has been used for the prevention of syphilis in herbal medicine. In addition, it has diuretic and antibacterial effects, and it is the ultimate purifier of blood. It will treat anemia, impotence in men, herpes, and other STDs, Dr. Sebi said.

Yellow dock root herb

Yellow dock, of Eurasian roots, is a flowering herb. It is rich in vitamins, iron, oxalic acid, and potassium. We should eat the leaves, if not too ripe, so the seeds and the roots turn bitter. To treat anemia, it has been used in herbal medicine. It is a detoxifier and blood purifier, especially for the liver, but also for the gallbladder. It increases the production of bile, which implies improved digestion. To help us remove the waste in the digestive tract sooner, it promotes bowel movement and raises the amount of urination to help us eliminate all pollutants.

Bladderwrack

Bladderwrack is a seaweed found in 1811 and used in iodine because of its high quality. Beta-carotene, zeaxanthin, volatile oils, calcium, paste, and other minerals are also high in it. Since it has anticoagulant properties, it should be prevented before surgery. It is used for thyroid gland enhancement and as a cure for cellulite and obesity in western medicine. Rheumatism and rheumatoid arthritis can also be alleviated by it. Bladderwrack powder is full of minerals that help remove contaminants from our skin, so we get rid of wrinkles, accumulation of extra water, and dryness. It also allows one to monitor the activity of the thyroid and reduce inflammation in the joints.

Kelp

Kelp is a seaweed that is mainly found on the coasts of Europe, Greenland, and North America. It is rich in iodine and phlorotannins, and is moderately high in vitamins and minerals in the diet. It is used to control the activity of the thyroid. Kelp tea encourages one to extract mucus from the body. This is why Dr. Sebi encourages us to use his flakes of organic kelp. Organic granules of kelp help us promote and regulate metabolism in the thyroid gland. They can also be used to reinforce our circulatory system, reduce the risk of heart failure and strokes, and maintain healthy bones and teeth. Thanks to its cancer-fighting benefits, it is still useful.

Irish moss tea

Irish moss is a red algae species that grows on the European and North American coasts. It is rich in vitamins, potassium, and minerals. Yet it's low in protein and fat. It is the only natural source of thyroid hormones and helps us extract our body's extra mucus. It is used in herbal medicine to heal sore throats and chest congestion.

Sting nettle leaf

Nettle leaf is a flowering plant of European origins that has been used for millennia in traditional medicines. It is relatively high in carbohydrates, proteins, and low in fat. A-linolenic acid (a valuable omega-3 acid) is also contained in it. It has been used since ancient times as a diuretic laxative in medicine. The herb is now used as an astringent, tonic, anti-rheumatic, anti-allergenic, decongestant, stimulant, and anti-spasmodic kidney cleanser. Diabetes and cancer are few of the diseases cured today. A great blood purifier, diuretic, astringent for UTI (urinary tract infections), and kidney stones are the sting nettle root in powder. It is also used for allergy, anemia, diabetes, hypertension, internal bleeding, osteoarthritis, and lung congestion. It is a remarkable tonic, often used for its anti-aging effects and wound healing.

Milk thistle

Milk thistle, now found all over the world, is a herb of Eurasian roots. It is a substantial silymarin, making it the ideal herb for the wellbeing of the liver. Cirrhosis, hepatitis, gallbladder diseases, and jaundice can be treated here. Scientific data is available for increased liver function and reduced deaths in people with liver disease after milk thistle is ingested.

Cleavers

Cleavers are of Eurasian descent, used in some countries for their edible leaves and seeds, but considered dangerous. It has a high concentration of iridoid glycosides, alkaloids, citric acid, flavonoids and coumarins. It is used as a diuretic and lymphatic tonic in medicine, and is also a beneficial blood purifier. It lets us cleanse urinary stones as a diuretic and treat urinary infections. For the lymphatic system, cleavers provide a cleansing action that helps us treat diseases like arthritis and psoriasis.

Red clover

The red clover is a herb of Eurasian origin, now cultivated all over the world, with edible flowers and leaves. Coumestrol and isoflavone are high in this drug. It can be used in the treatment of cancer, elevated cholesterol, cough, pneumonia, indigestion, bronchitis, and STDs. In people with coagulation problems, it is safer to prevent it. It is considered a cleansing agent for blood. It is used by women to ease menopause, breast pain, and PMS (premenstrual syndrome) symptoms. For skin sores, burns, psoriasis, and certain skin cancers, skin instruments are used.

Blue vervain

Blue vervain is a herb which grows throughout North America naturally. For decades, it has been used in herbal medicine to relax the liver and other organs and to relieve the central nervous system. It is a tonic that can also be used to alleviate coughing congestion, to relieve coughs, to reduce fever, to relax the nerves, and to cleanse contaminants.

Shepherd's purse

It is a mustard-family flowering plant of Eurasian roots, used for fruit and medicine. There are antioxidant, anti-inflammatory and anti-mucous properties in the shepherd's purse. It is used as an astringent in urinary tract infections and also to minimize inflammation, shield us from ulcers, promote circulation, and boost urine production. Different illnesses, such as bleeding problems, diarrhea, urinary infections, low blood pressure, headaches, and kidney failure, may be managed using it. It can be added directly to the skin in the case of cuts and burns to soothe discomfort and facilitate healing. Scientific evidence of its impact on reducing tumor growth is scant.

Yarrow herb

Yarrow herb is a flowering plant that has a long history of herbal medicine use in temperate regions. It is rich in essential oils, salicylic acid, isovaleric acid, and flavonoids. For millennia, it has been used in traditional European and Asian medicine to heal wounds. To alleviate fever, relieve digestive problems, and heal wounds and burns, Native Americans used it for toothaches. It is the ultimate organ recovery plant, and it can also be used as a tonic for the venous system and mucous membranes of chronic urinary tract diseases. It is useful for throat pain, bleeding, urinary incontinence, and diabetes.

Chickweed

Chickweed is a flowering plant of Eurasian origin that has been used as a herbal remedy for decades. It may also be found in salads or other dishes, as a leaf vegetable. It has been used to treat itches, lung disorders, rheumatic symptoms, and arthritis in herbal medicine. It is now used as a diuretic and as demulcent because by creating a calming layer over it it alleviates the discomfort and irritation of the mucous membrane. It is used by dietitians and herbalists because it suppresses cravings.

Valerian root

Valerian is a flowering plant that has been used in medicine since ancient times with European roots. It is rich in alkaloids, iridoids, flavanones, and isovaleric acid. Used to treat insomnia and other sleep disturbances, it is an important sedative. It is also used for conditions similar to anxiety, such as nervous asthma, disease panic, and paranoia, although no trials have produced definitive findings. Some people use it to combat depression, mild tremors, CFS (chronic fatigue syndrome), and ADHD (attention deficit-hyperactivity disorder). Women also use valerian to soothe menstrual cramps and all conditions associated with menopause, to relieve hot sweats and anxiety.

Damiana leaves

Damiana has aromatic flowers and leaves with a fiery scent and taste, and is a Central American shrub. It is rich in flavonoids, glycosides, damianine, beta-carotene, and moderately high in fatty acids and caffeine. It is used for heightened vitality, moderate depression, menstrual pain, impotence, and sexual arousal in western medicine.

Chaparral

Chaparral is a plant that spreads in the Americas and is medicinal. It has been used for treating STDs, measles, dysmenorrhea, chickenpox, and snake bites in herbal medicine. It is now used to treat bronchitis, arthritis, intestinal cramps, colds, and chronic skin conditions to relieve rheumatic and stomach pains. It has also been used for problems with the liver, inflammation of the gall bladder and urinary tract, kidney stones, and diarrhea. For rheumatism, inflammation, mild burns, back pain, and skin diseases, skin application is used.

Foods to Avoid

Some ingredients, mostly packaged foods, animal-based or formulated with leavening agents, are not included in Dr. Sebi's Diet. Also certain seedless fruits are forbidden. We have to pay heed to what nutrients we will require when we have to work with a diet. They range from vitamins and minerals to other foods, including fatty acids such as iron, calcium, and omega-3. However, if you also mix your recipes, you can get the most nutrients from the sources dependent on plants.

Sugar

You can use sweeteners such as pure agave syrup (from cacti) or date sugar (from dried dates) instead of sugar.

Salt

You might use powdered, granulated seaweed or pure sea salt instead of refined salt. No things that are GMO! The removal of pesticides and other contaminants applied to manufactured or genetically modified crops is crucial. If it is not normal, in the long run, it would affect us.

The primary foods to be avoided are:

Meat of any kind

Food is high in water, proteins and vitamins (755), but poor in calories, carbohydrates and nutritional minerals. Based on race, sex, age, and other aspects, even though the amount of fat is minimal, the bad side is that all meat produces cholesterol, which affects our overall health. Nutritionists warn us to steer as far away from meat as possible, in particular red meat, so there is a greater chance of cancer, heart disease and obesity for its users. Items made from processed beef, Dr. Sebi said, are much worse. Processed meat also contains dietary additives in addition to the high amount of animal-based proteins that only improve the acidic state of our body.

Seafood and fish

The high content of omega-3 fatty acids that are suitable for our brain, heart and digestive system makes fish and seafood popular. In specific, fish and shrimp are the main components of the Mediterranean diet. Nevertheless, we must bear in mind that it is still a very large reservoir of natural or human-made hazardous materials, such as aquatic chemicals, bacteria, pollutants, and other poisons.

Dairy products

Dairy goods are used in different ways globally and are detrimental to persons with lactose intolerance. Cholesterol, potassium, and saturated fats are used, which can lead to an elevated risk of heart failure, calcification of the coronary artery, and other complications. Despite certain misconceptions, milk and other dairy products do not induce mucus formation, so do not intensify the symptoms of asthma. Only for ethical considerations as to how the animals are treated and how dairy products are made are they avoided by vegans.

Eggs

Eggs are yet another abundant source of proteins originating from plants. Fat, calcium, vitamins, water (75 percent), and cholesterol are also high in them. Eggs can be stopped to the fullest degree possible, according to Dr. Sebi and other nutritionists. Egg intake is limited to a limit of two eggs a week with virtually every diet, but Dr. Sebi urges us to put them aside. Heart diseases, such as strokes, lung disease, coronary artery disease, myocardial infarction, and type 2 diabetes, are more likely to occur.

Wheat

Wheat is an Eastern-origin tree, now planted for its seeds internationally. It is rich in dietary nutrients, sugars, folate, and moderately high in proteins and selenium, but low in fat. For bread, crackers, spaghetti, breakfast cereals, biscuits, and some alcoholic beverages, it is used as the main ingredient. A diet rich in grains, vegetables and fruits is bound to help us sustain a healthier weight, reduce the risk of heart disease, and certain forms of cancer, most nutritionists say. The biggest issue with wheat is that it produces high levels of gluten, a major concern not just for bloating, but also for neurological disorders, fibromyalgia, nausea, and psychological conditions for those who suffer from gluten-related diseases.

Corn

Corn is an American-origin cereal grain, world-famous for its sweet flavor, but most of all, for popcorn. It is high in water (76%), carbohydrates, a moderate dietary fiber source, minerals, but low in protein and fat. As it contains lipid transfer protein, Dr. Sebi urges us to keep it at bay. This protein causes allergic reactions, such as vomiting, mucous membrane swelling, diarrhea, and occasionally asthma.

Garlic

Garlic has a long tradition of use as food and medicine and is a close relative of the onion, of Asian roots. It is known to be a natural antibiotic. It has been used to cure arthritis, chronic cough, mosquito and snake bites, and antiseptic medications to prevent gangrene in conventional medicine. It includes flavonoids, saponins, and polysulfides. Carbohydrates, antioxidants, dietary fibre, fats, and fat are low in it. As its intake can lead to stomach pain, dizziness, allergic reactions, sweating, and bleeding, it is banned from our diet. It also contains the essential trace element selenium, which if ingested in excess, is poisonous.

Sugar

Sugar is high in sugars and low in dietary fiber, proteins, and fat. Sugar, widely used as an additive to processed foods, is a refined food. It is therefore really dangerous to our welfare. Most nutritionists argue that it is most possible that its heavy use would create addiction. We recognize that this is associated to an elevated risk of type 2 diabetes, tooth loss, obesity, cardiovascular disease, metabolic syndrome, and even dementia. As mentioned earlier, it is only natural sugar from fruit, vegetables, or agave syrup and date sugar that is better used.

Fast foods

The most friendly and quick to produce foods are fast foods, and let's confess, the ultimate sort of food that is eye-catching and mouth-watering. In our new, hectic times in particular! We're always in a hurry, always rushing around college, families, and other everyday problems. It's not yet time for any of us to enjoy at least three meals a day. You're great if you can quietly have dinner with your family or friends! The remedy? Of course, fast food. Junk food and nothing more, so what can we do to make this change? It is difficult to start changing your eating habits, particularly when you have to eat a diet, just as in our case! Not only with a nose twist or a finger snap. With lots and lots of patience and the steady incorporation into your diet of good ingredients! Unfortunately, obesity, elevated levels of cholesterol, and even depression are often correlated with quick snacks. For the right reasons!

Processed foods

Perhaps worst is processed foods. To make them taste healthier, to be enticing to consumers, easy to eat on the go and for longer shelf lives, all kinds of ingredients are used. Another bad point is that there is little or no whole food in them; they are just micronutrient fortified. In the long term, it would be more difficult for our body to keep up with toxic elements with all these chemicals, sweeteners, refining acids, flavours and preservatives. There is a greater chance of contracting cardiovascular illnesses, such as obesity, diabetes, heart disease, asthma and certain cancers, owing to the intake of processed foods.

Seedless fruits

All fruits which contain no mature seeds are seedless fruits. Because their consumption is simpler, they are economically important. Watermelons, onions, tomatoes, and citrus fruits fall under this grou

Chapter five: Alkaline diet

Health advantages of a diet focused on alkaline plants

The alkaline diet is perfect whether you are a vegetarian, vegan, or looking to step in this direction. Although all food plans should be founded around a solid vegetable and fruit basis, one of the better choices for adhering to this way of eating is a plant-based diet. Not all vegan or plant-based diets are alkaline; it is possible to process a number of foods that are free from animal products and contain acidic components, while certain 'acidic' fruits and vegetables become alkaline once digested. Soy is one of the most helpful, nutrient-rich foods for an alkaline diet. As with tofu, tempeh, miso and other soy-based ingredients, soybeans (edamame beans) are a perfect snack on their own. Look for organic, safe alternatives when buying soy products, and skip preservatives as far as possible.

Why choose a diet based on plants?

From eliminating meat in your diet overall to introducing one or two "meat-free days" per week, there are several reasons to switch to a plant-based diet. This will take a big change if the current diet is very meat-heavy, so it is best not to turn from red meats immediately to complete veganism. Instead of canned or refined options, veganism or vegetarianism works well when whole, raw ingredients are selected. In the promotion of meat-free processed snacks and condiments, a lot of publicity is involved, although many of these may include calories, large levels of salt, artificial colour, additives, and other harmful ingredients. To encourage a plant-based diet, there is a lot of study and the high level of alkaline in many fruits and vegetables means a good combination for the alkaline-based diet:

·   The focus is on natural foods as a whole which simplifies the buying process and the variety of food for your diet. As the emphasis will be on vegetarian-based eating, without meat as an alternative, and little or no dairy, this also makes meal preparation and planning much simpler.

·   As vegetables and fruits are digested and used much more easily than meat and dairy products, a plant-based diet can help with weight loss. Vegetarian meals often have less calories, except though the total serving size is the same or close to a meal, including meat.

·   It is a great accomplishment to reach your target weight, and keeping weight is another challenge. With plant-based feeding, this can be done even more easily, as there are not only limits on the intake of meat and dairy, but also on refined foods that also contain by-products of meat (gelatin) and a high level of preservatives and artificial flavors.

·   Soy is a major staple of a diet focused on vegetables. In soy products, the amount of calcium, protein, iron and nutrients is equal to beef and a proportion of the calories and fat. Soy in most grocery stores is still relatively cheap and easy to find. In almost every type of meal, tofu, tempeh, and edamame beans are common ways to enjoy soy.

·   It can mitigate or remove food sensitivities to dairy and meat products by enjoying a plant-based diet, since they are no longer part of the diet. Other food allergies or sensitivities may be less of a factor, since digestion becomes better and wellbeing improves overall, until a greater pH equilibrium is formed throughout the body.

·   There are various health benefits from a plant-based diet, especially vegan, where both meat by-products and dairy foods are fully excluded. Type 2 diabetes, among many other disorders, from strengthening heart wellbeing and respiratory function to stopping cancer. Prevention is a significant consideration in which a plant-based diet is preferred, since it is easy to prevent certain conditions and diseases in the first place.

In an Alkaline Diet, the value of Soy

There are a number of research and observations on soy that result in promising results and advantages of consuming soy on the risks of increasing estrogen and the effect on your health when it comes to soy. Overall, for any diet, soy is a healthy choice, particularly for vegan diets focused on plants that exclude all meat products. Some substitutes may be considered by people with allergies of soy and soy-based goods to effectively stick to a vegan meal schedule. With the following benefits, soy is a healthy choice for most individuals:

1.   Elevated in protein. Soy will fill your diet with just as much, if not more, protein than beef. Your body can consume more than the necessary daily protein in tandem with a healthy diet that includes fresh vegetables and fruits.

2.   Low in cholesterol: Cholesterol, saturated, and trans fats are low in plant-based diets, making them a healthy choice for good cardiovascular health and a way to reduce cardiac disease.

3.   It's rich in fiber. Soy is very rich in nutrition, as are all vegetables and fruits. By converting to soy from beef, you will not only fulfill your regular protein, calcium, and iron needs, you will also get a decent dose of fiber for each meal, which improves metabolism and preserves weight at a stable, sustainable amount.

4.   Few soy products also contain vitamin B12 and other nutrients considered only present in meat and meat-related products. In order to satisfy nutritional needs, fermented soy, such as miso and tempeh, contains an adequate quantity of B12.

5.   As it is fortified, vitamin D is also an ingredient in dairy milk, but this can also be present in different soy products. Although it takes just a small amount of this vitamin, it's essential to make it a part of your diet.

6.   In many shapes, textures, and flavors, Soy products come. For starters, soft tofu varieties can be used for making puddings, cakes, and smoothies. Firm tofu and tempeh can be marinated with some mixture of vegetables and ingredients, and grilled, cooked, or sautéed. Soy milk can be used in cereals, in smoothies, milkshakes, and as a cooling drink as a better alternative to dairy.

7.   They're easy to eat. Although some individuals have reported bloating and minor soy digestion problems, in general, it is easy for the body to absorb food and break down nutrients.

Alternatives for a Plant-Based Diet to Soy

There are several options to choose from if soy-based foods are not an option for your plant-based diet. These foods contain high levels of protein, calcium, and iron present in meat and milk products, including:

Coconut-cultured yogurt:

Vegan, coconut-based yogurt, similar to dairy yogurt, is produced by cultivating coconut bacterial culture to produce a food of the same texture, nutrients, and taste as dairy yogurt.

Vegan cheese:

Most vegan cheese types are soy-based, while vegetables and vegetable oils are made from an increasing range of plant-based cheeses. The advantages of vegan cheese include a flavor and texture close to that of traditional milk cheese. Unlike soy-based goods, vegetable-based cheese appears to melt easier, making this variation a preferred choice for grilled vegan cheese and Mac-and-cheese dishes.

Milk from peanuts, cashews, and coconuts:

At almost every grocery store and local restaurant, there are many non-dairy milk alternatives available. In addition to other nut-based forms of milk, including cashew milk, almond milk is becoming almost as popular as soymilk. For a sweet, nut-like flavor that works well in recipes, smoothies, and with cereal, some varieties have a mixture of almond and coconut milk, or cashew and almond. More individuals are ditching milk and cream for their coffee and tea for non-dairy alternatives as well. Other options include milk derived from hemp and corn.

Nut Butters:

An excellent source of protein and nutrition is peanuts, almonds, and other forms of nut butter. Prior to a workout or a busy day, only one or two spoons of these butters will have a strong nutritional boost.

Other Alternatives to Soy:

Instead of tofu and other soy foods, nuts and seeds can be added to stir-fry dishes and salads to increase the protein and calcium content. For baking and preparing vegetarian meals, olive oil or coconut oil are also suitable options. Both oils have a neutral taste, which goes well for any product mix.

Alkaline Fruits

With natural sugars that can quickly replace the need for sweet sweets and refined foods, fruits are an excellent source of vitamins, nutrition, and energy. We prefer to pick from a small circle or category of fruits when we shop for fruits that we are acquainted and happy with. The range or restrictions on what fruit we purchase can depend on what is in season, how much of a budget we have to work with and our preferences. Bananas, apples, oranges, and berries seem to be the most common, and are tasty and simple to eat for a good cause. When they are in the peak season, apples are best during autumn and are available in several varieties that differ in texture, flavor, and appearance. It's the best time to eat new fruits during the summer months, such as tomatoes, bananas and melons. During winter or colder seasons, whether you buy local, fresh fruits become less affordable. Another choice to explore is frozen fruits. As they last longer and can be used at any time, they are just as safe and more convenient. It is necessary to avoid canned foods, including vegetables or fruits, since they contain extra salt and sugar, along with other additives.

What fruits have a high alkaline content?

There is a substantial amount of alkaline in all fruits, making them all good options for an alkaline diet. The proportions differ depending on the fruit, where the alkaline content is either medium, moderate or heavy. Some fruits containing acidic properties, such as tomatoes and citrus fruits, are converted to alkaline once digested, while others contain high amounts of alkaline before consumption:

- Raspberries, blackberries, and strawberries. Because of their high level of vitamin C and antioxidants, berries are a perfect alternative for an alkaline diet.

- Nectarines are rich in alkaline content, like peaches, and make a perfect snack on their own or in a fruit salad.

- Not only are watermelons rich in alkaline, they also have a decent proportion of potassium and fiber. They are an excellent option for a snack and when more readily available, exceptionally refreshing during the summer season.

- Apples have more of an alkaline quantity that is more intermediate to heavy, but they have a lot of nutrients at any time of year that make them a favorite snack. For a number of recipes, they may be savoured raw, stewed, or fried. Also, apples are naturally delicious, making them suitable for desserts.

- Bananas are rich in carbohydrate, potassium, and carry a great deal of energy into only one serving. In reality, up to 90 minutes of energy can be provided by one banana; a simple and fast snack before a run, walk, or bike trip.

- Similar to grapes, cherries are rich in fiber and alkaline. They still advocate continuity and balanced metabolism. Are there fruits that can be avoided? For an alkaline diet, nearly all fruits are excellent alternatives that make it easier to adopt the diet.

Chapter Six: Who is Dr. Sebi

INTRODUCTION OF THE DR. SEBI TREATMENTS AND CURES"

The healing and care of Dr. Sebi is focused on the power of the human body to self-heal. Beyond all doubt, biologists have already proved that the human body has a phenomenal capacity to combat any type of illness. In addition to the adverse impact of air pollutants, the medications we take for symptomatic relaxation and the junk food we consume in vast amounts contribute to the production of many chronic diseases, which in the Western world are increasingly becoming the leading cause of death. The body's defenses and disease-fighting abilities are compromised by poor eating habits and dependence on medications. The curing of Dr. Sebi is rooted in herbs and barks: the best way to healthily and spontaneously strengthen the immunity of the body. Not only because of the health benefits, but for the overall well-being that it fosters, you should consider adhering to his values and diet. But let's explore first what the diagnosis and care of Dr. Sebi is all about and then we will move on to how his herbal cure works for diseases.

This diet is solely based on the African biomineral equilibrium theory and was formulated using the study of the herbalist Alfredo Darrington Bowman, best known as Dr. Sebi, who was self-taught. He developed his diet, without focusing on traditional Western medications, for everyone who wants to treat or avoid chronic diseases and improve their general health. The disease is the product of mucus production in a certain location in the body, according to Dr. Sebi. An accumulation of mucus in the lungs, for example, is pneumonia, while diabetes is the excess mucus within the pancreas. He notes that in an alkaline environment, viruses will <u>not</u> occur and start to emerge as soon as the body becomes too acidic.

Therefore you are assured to preserve the normal alkaline state of your body and detoxify your disease-riddled body by strictly following his weight loss strategy and using his unique dietary supplements and herbs. A detailed list of everyday fruits, culms, beans, nuts, berries, oils, and herbs is included in the weight reduction program. As animal products are not allowed, the Balanced Eating Plan of Dr. Sebi is known to be a vegan diet. Sebi said that in order for the body to regenerate on its own for the remainder of your life, you must regularly follow your diet. For several years, Dr. Sebi, a herbal practitioner, has used his alkaline plants and diets to treat herpes and chronic illnesses, and this can be attested to by the testimonials of his patients, including some very high profile ones.

Who is Dr. Sebi, and what ideology does he have?

Alfredo Bowman is the man behind the Dr. Sebi Diet. He's a self-proclaimed herbalist and healer from Honduras who uses food to improve his health. While he is now gone, in the 21st century, he has a lot of supporters. He has claimed to treat all kinds of diseases using herbs and a strict vegan diet, because of his holistic approach. Before coming to New York City, he founded a rehab facility in his home country, where he expanded his practice and grew his clientele, to name a few to Michael Jackson, John Travolta, Eddie Murphy, and Steven Seagal.

Although he calls himself Dr. Sebi, he does not have a degree in medicine or a Ph.D. In addition, multiple diseases such as sickle cell anemia, lupus, leukemia, and HIV-AIDS have been believed to be treated by the diet. This led to many problems particularly because he practiced medicine without a license and his exorbitant arguments. While he was convicted of practicing without a license, he was cleared because of a lack of evidence in the early 1990s. He was however, told to avoid making suggestions that

HIV-AIDS could be treated by his diet. Although there are disputes surrounding his reputation, his alkaline vegan diet has so many advantages that it is still popular up to this day.

The Alkaline Eating Diet of Dr.Sebi

Dr. Sebi assumed that various kinds of diseases could be caused by acidity and mucus. The build-up of mucus in the lungs, for example, will contribute to pneumonia. He noted that it may help to detoxify the body by consuming some kinds of food and avoiding those like the plague. It can also get the body to an alkaline condition that can reduce the chance of certain kinds of diseases being created.

The cells can be rejuvenated by turning the blood alkaline, and can effectively remove toxins. In addition, he states that in an atmosphere that is alkaline, infections cannot occur. What other plant-based diets bank on is his theory of making the body more alkaline.

This specific diet depends on the consumption of certain types of vitamins as well as consuming a selection of approved foods. Dr. Sebi noted that for the body to cure itself this diet should be practiced regularly for the remainder of the life. The Dr. Sebi Diet is plant-based, although there are certain distinctions in this diet and the plant-based diet in general, unlike most plant-based diets. Here is a compiled list of what separates a plant-based diet from the Dr. Sebi Diet.

The cells can be rejuvenated by turning the blood alkaline, and can effectively remove toxins. In addition, he states that in an atmosphere that is alkaline, infections cannot occur. What other plant-based diets bank on is his theory of making the body more alkaline. This specific diet depends on the consumption of certain types of vitamins as well as consuming a selection of approved foods. Dr. Sebi noted that for the body to cure itself this diet should be practiced regularly for the remainder of the life. The Dr. Sebi Diet is plant-based, although there are certain distinctions in this diet and the plant-based diet in general, unlike most plant-based diets. Here is a compiled list of what separates a plant-based diet from the Dr. Sebi Diet.

No refined foods are considered processed: tofu, veggie burgers, textured vegetable protein, canned fruits, canned vegetables, oil, soy sauce, and other condiments. The Dr. Sebi Diet allows dieters to eat unadulterated foods. As long as they are made from plant-based materials, certain plant-based diets do promote the use of refined foods.

No wheat products permitted: You are not allowed to ingest wheat and wheat products such as bread, biscuits, and others under this diet regimen because they are not naturally produced grains. Amaranth beans, wild rice, and triticale, to name a few, contain naturally growing crops.

The requirement to stick to the food list: plant-based diets in general are not so stringent when it comes to the food that dieters are required to consume (unless you strictly adopt a rigid plant-based regimen such as the keto diet based on plants). The Dr. Sebi Diet, however, allows dieters to consume only foods specified in the dietary guide.

Drink a gallon of water daily: the most hydrating liquid on the planet is water. Dieters are expected by the Dr. Sebi Diet to drink 1 gallon of water daily or more. Moreover, since these beverages are extremely acidic, tea and coffee can be avoided.

Taking Dr. Sebi's supplements: This unique diet regimen would require you to take patented supplements an hour before taking the prescription if you are taking some medicine for a certain health problem.

Teachings and Approaches by Dr. Sebi

As the amount of toxins and mucus accumulation rose, Dr. Sebi suggested that the body is at the point of being vulnerable to contracting diseases. He concluded that people suffering from multiple diseases and those involved in disease prevention should still consume an alkaline diet, keeping in mind that it becomes free of bacteria as the body avoids the elevated volume of acidic substances and mucus. He also indicated that body cleaning and detoxification is a necessary and important method required to cope with any type of illness in the body. Body detoxification tends to eliminate mucus accumulated in the liver, lungs, and many other organs of the body and also helps to remove excess acidic compounds, leaving the body free of disease-causing diseases. Dr. Sebi has made use of herbs that are important for the body to be re-energized and revitalized. When there is a change in your health, the organs of the body operate well and this means that the body is devoid of diseases.

Dr. Sebi Food Classification; Dr. Sebi has divided food into six groups. All classifications are:

- Narcotics.

- Foods that are genetically engineered.

- Food hybrids.

- Dead groceries.

- Food for life.

- About raw ingredients.

He concluded that the first four food types in this category are not a go-area because they do more harm than damage to the body. A build-up of acids and mucus in the body may affect these foods. However since the nutrient quality of them is not lost in any way, the last two forms of food are the best forms of food he has listed as good. For example, the necessary amount of nutrients present in them has been lost by foods that are extensively fried, hybridized, and modified. Therefore the opposite is the case instead of having advantages for the body. Raw foods, however are excellent for building good health, especially vegetables, fruits, and herbs. Details regarding The Diet of Dr. Sebi. Dr. Sebi's diets are plant-based and electric-based diets. The diets of Dr. Sebi are African bio-mineral diets that help dieters fight illnesses. The diet is also used to combat many diseases (prophylaxis) and helps to improve the immune system. It is said to tolerate any virus that sneaks in while the body is immuno-compromised. The diet of Dr. Sebi is also helpful for individuals who love to live a healthy life by staying safe and lean. His diet wasn't made from heaven; because of the love of modified, industrialized, refined, and hybridized ingredients, they are typical foods we ignore.

The diet of Dr. Sebi includes vegetables, fruits, rice, nuts, herbal teas, sweeteners dependent on herbs, and seeds. This diet would not help those who cherish animal products as it does not promote foods that are made from animals. Both pathogens grow well in the atmosphere, according to Dr. Sebi, keeping them relaxed, such as acid, mucus excess, and poisonous surroundings. Infections will find it so difficult to prosper when the body is in a limy condition, and when it is in an acidic state, the opposite is the case. The acidic portion of the body thus allows illnesses to spread and thrive. He further claimed that the buildup of extra mucus in the body increases the susceptibility of developing an infection as the mucus fills the blood stream and quickly hinders the blood flow. He claimed that for you to enjoy your wellbeing, the extra mucus must be eliminated. The infections are naturally eliminated as the mucus is removed by either detoxification or washing. Dr. Sebi's diets have been shown to be successful by those who really enjoy them. By taking the body back to its natural state, diets re-energize and revitalize the body. The recovery of many people suffering from hair loss and many other common ailments did not arise due to the drugs they took, but due to the self-healing that took place in the body due to the alkaline diet of Dr. Sebi.

Nutritional Diet Lists of Dr. Sebi

Nutritional food lists from Dr. Sebi are listed below:

Diets for Vegetables

Dulse, Garbanzo Beans, Arame, Wild Arugula, Avocado, Cucumber, Dandelion Leaves, Amaranth, Watercress, Tomatillo, Turnip Greens, Wakame, Lettuce, Olives, Purslane Verdolaga, Squash, Okra, Hijiki, Nopales, Nori, Zucchini and Onions, Izote flower and leaf, Kale, Mushrooms other than Shitake, Bell Pepper, Chayote, Cherry and Plum Tomato,

Diets on fruits

Dates, Figs, Plums, Strawberries, Onions, Pears, Limes, Pineapple, Tomatoes, Raisins, Papayas, Melons, and Currants: Peaches, Orange, Soft Jelly Coconuts, Cantaloupe, Prickly Pear, Cherries, Prunes, Bananas,

Diets for Alkaline Grains

Kamut, Tef, Spelt, Fonio, Wild Rice, Amaranth, Quinoa, and Rye.

Products of Alkaline Sugar

- Date Sugar.

- Agave Syrup from cactus (100% Pure).

Herbs Item

Dill, Onion powder, Basil, Pure sea salt, Oregano, and Cayenne.

Spices and Diets for Seasoning

Bay Leaf, Cayenne, Sweet Basil, Garlic, Onion Powder, Sage, Oregano, Ground Granulated Seaweed, and Tarragon. Dill, Achiote, Habanero, Savory, Basil, Thyme, Pure Sea Salt,

Items of Herbal Tea

Elderberry, Tila, Burdock, Ginger, Fennel, Chamomile, Red Raspberry

Benefits of Dr. Sebi's Medication

The Dr. Sebi Diet presents dieters with a number of advantages. Although it is recognized that the foods prescribed by this diet decrease inflammation, there are other advantages that you can gain from adopting the Dr. Sebi Diet.

Can aid in weight loss

While this diet regimen is not meant for weight loss, it will benefit individuals who wish to lose weight. Studies suggest that individuals who eat an unrestricted whole plant-based diet report substantial compa weight loss. In this diet, the way people lose weight depends on the high fiber and low-calorie foods you are encouraged to consume. Most foods advocated by the Dr. Sebi Diet are low in calories, except for avocados, almonds, beans, and oil. Yet they are not only calorie-dense, but also rich in fiber and minerals, even though you eat nuts and seeds.

Colon Health is Higher

Because this eating regimen promotes the ingestion of significant amounts of fruits and vegetables, it also benefits the health of the colon. Fiber-rich diets can help facilitate balanced digestion, but there is no constipation for those who adopt the Dr. Sebi Diet.

Controlling appetite

While many people claim that this diet is very restricting in terms of the number of calories that a single individual takes in, there are research that show that this diet can help regulate appetite. A high degree of satiety can be provided by the high fiber in your diet which can help you feel satisfied for much longer.

The Better Microbiota Gut

The second brain is the stomach. Not only can the enzymes and molecules released by the bacteria in the gut influence your wellbeing, but also your daily mood. The types of molecules that bacteria release into the bloodstream are often affected by what you bring within your system. The amount of food you often eat will influence the type of bacteria in your stomach as well. Studies, for example, indicate that intake of greasy, oily, and refined foods can lead to a decrease in good microorganisms and stimulate the body's growth of bad bacteria.

Inflammation Minimized

While inflammation is one of the first line of protection of the body signaling the existence of infection and illnesses, inflammation of chronic low doses may also be bad for the body. In reality, chronic inflammation can lead to many forms of illnesses, including diabetes, stroke, and even cancer. Thus, fruit and vegetable-rich diets are related to decreased inflammation caused by oxidative stress. In contrast to those that consume animal products, studies that look at people eating plant-based diets have a 31 percent lower risk of developing heart disorders and cancer. He developed this diet for someone who instinctively wishes to avoid or treat some sickness. Without using chemical drugs, it can also increase your general health. The hypothesis of Dr. Sebi is that because of so much mucus piling up in a certain region of the body, all infections are induced. You get pneumonia because you get so much mucus in your lungs. This causes diabetes if you have too much mucus in your pancreas. He assumes that in an alkaline climate, any illness would not occur, but if the body is too acidic, it will happen. While inflammation is one of the first line of protection of the body signaling the existence of infection and illnesses, inflammation of chronic low doses may also be bad for the body. In reality, chronic inflammation can lead to many forms of illnesses, including diabetes, stroke, and even cancer. Thus, fruit and vegetable-rich diets are related to decreased inflammation caused by oxidative stress. In contrast to those that consume animal products, studies that look at people eating plant-based diets have a 31 percent lower risk of developing heart disorders and cancer. He developed this diet for someone who instinctively wishes to avoid or treat some sickness. Without using chemical drugs, it can also increase your general health.

The hypothesis of Dr. Sebi is that because of so much mucus piling up in a certain region of the body, all infections are induced. You get pneumonia because you get so much mucus in your lungs. This causes diabetes if you have too much mucus in your pancreas. He assumes that in an alkaline climate, any illness would not occur, but if the body is too acidic, it will happen. Many people believe that by consuming his compounds, his diet preserved their health, and the herbal approach to curing the body performed better than any medicinal approach ever did. Long after his death, you can find plenty of his insights on YouTube about herbal therapy and dietary compounds that help foster and encourage healthy living. His lifestyle provides plenty of health benefits. The key one is that it will stimulate weight loss because it limits packaged foods, and you can consume more unprocessed, plant-based meals. This diet is full of whole vegetables and fruits that are full of fiber, minerals, vitamins, and plant compounds. Oxidative stress and decreased inflammation are associated with diets containing fruits and vegetables, along with shielding you from most diseases. Meatless diets have been related to lower rates of obesity and heart disease. Foods that are rich in fibre and low in calories are also promoted. Consuming fruits and vegetables daily will help shield the body from diseases and decrease inflammation. If you can turn from your usual diet full of fast carbohydrates, saturated fats, processed sugars and grains to the diet of Dr. Sebi, raising your consumption of wheat, vegetables and fruits while getting rid of pork and beef can potentially help you shed some weight, decreasing your risk of elevated cholesterol, high blood pressure, type 2 diabetes, heart disease and cancer. Many people consume so much salt, and this diet will reduce this level significantly. This will help decrease your blood pressure, in exchange, and this increases your risk of heart attack and stroke. In one report, individuals who ate seven servings of fruits and vegetables a day were 25 to 31 percent less likely to develop heart disease and cancer. They don't eat enough produce for most Americans. It was estimated that 9.3 to 12.2 percent met all of their recommended daily intake of fruits and vegetables during 2017. Dr. Sebi's diet promotes healthier fats such as plant oils, beans and nuts to be consumed along with fiber-rich whole grain. There is a lower chance of contracting heart disease from these foods. Any diet that reduces refined foods will help to increase the consistency of your diet.

Dr. Sebi STD Treatments

STDs are also fairly common, associated with sexually transmitted infections, even though there are well-known ways to avoid them. There are several diseases that fall under the STD group which are transmitted by sexual contact, but can be spread in other ways. Trichomoniasis, syphilis, certain forms of hepatitis, gonorrhoea, genital warts, genital herpes, chlamydia, and HIV are the most common STDs. STDs were referred to as venereal disorders at one time. They are some of the most common diseases that are infectious. An incurable STD has been diagnosed by over 65 million Americans. 20 million new cases occur per year, and about half of them occur in individuals aged 15 to 24. These will all have long-term effects. There are extreme diseases which need to be treated. Any of them are considered incurable and such as HIV, can be fatal. Information on how to defend yourself will be given by learning more about these diseases. Via genital, vaginal and anal intercourse, STDs may be transmitted. Via contact with a moist or damp material, such as toilet seats, wet clothes, or towels, trichomoniasis may be transmitted, although it is often transmitted through sexual intercourse. Individuals who are at increased risk of STDs include:

- Those that have a single sexual partner .

- Those that swap sex for money or drugs.

- Those that exchange drug-use needles.

- Those that, during intercourse, don't use condoms.

- Those who have sex with a person who has had multiple partners.

The two STDs that are chronic diseases that medical medicine does not treat but can only treat are Herpes and HIV. Hepatitis B can become chronic at times. Unfortunately, once it has impaired your reproductive organs, heart, vision, or other organs, you often may not figure out if you have an STD. The immune system will also be damaged by STDs, leaving you susceptible to other diseases. Pelvic inflammatory disorder can be caused by chlamydia and gonorrhea and this can leave people unable to conceive. It is also capable of murdering you. The kid could face permanent harm if an STD were passed on to a child, or it could kill them.

Causes of STDs

In terms of clinical medicine, both forms of infection induce STDs. Bacteria include Syphilis, gonorrhea, and Chlamydia. All are infectious, such as hepatitis B, vaginal warts, genital herpes, and HIV. Trichomoniasis produces parasites. In vaginal secretions, blood semen, and in certain instances, saliva, the STD germs remain inside. Most species can spread by oral, anal, or vaginal penetration, but some can spread directly by skin-to-skin contact, such as with genital warts and genital herpes. Hepatitis B may be acquired by exchanging personal products, such as razors or toothbrushes.

Prevention

The most apparent move for STDs in recovery is not to get one in the first place. The first tip people offer to prevent STDs is not to have sex with people with genital discharge, rash, sores, or other signs, or at least to stop sex with them. The only time you can have casual sex is if you and your wife are only having sex with each other, and in the last six months, all reports have been negative for STDs. Otherwise you'll have to make sure:

Whenever you are having sex, use condoms. Make sure it is one that is water-based if you use a lubricant. Condoms for the whole act of sex should be included. Bear in mind when it comes to avoiding pregnancy or illness, condoms are not 100% successful. However, if you use them the right way, they are very powerful.

- Stop swapping towels or undergarments.

- Since and before you have sex, bathe.

- You will get vaccinations for a couple of STDs, especially Hep B and HPV, if you are comfortable with vaccination.

- Make sure that you are HIV-tested.

- Please get treatment if you misuse alcohol or medications. Getting unprotected sex is more common for persons who are under the influence.

- Finally, the only 100 percent successful means of avoiding STDs is to abstain from sex altogether.

There was a suggestion that by destroying the pathogens that triggered them, using a condom with nonoxynol-9 would eliminate STDs. New research has shown that this may end up irritating the cervix and vagina of the woman and may increase her chance of an STD. You are urged to avoid nonoxynol-9 condoms.

CHAPTER SEVEN: THE DR. SEBI HERPES CURE

Cure for Herpes

An alkaline-rich diet rich in vital nutrients can help get rid of the herpes virus in your body. This can be done by developing an ecosystem which can not facilitate the production of substance-causing diseases. In order to work to their optimal potential, the cells in the body require oxygen, but the chemicals and substances present in certain drugs and foods take the much-needed oxygen from the cells to survive. It needs proper washing of the body to heal the herpes virus, and the plant-based alkaline diet of Dr. Sebi does exactly that. It is important to note that herpes care relies on the kinds of food you consume and what you are feeding the body with.

You should stop consuming starchy foods and desserts. Eat salty, rather than sweet foods. Eat healthier vegetables such as zucchini, onions, squash, flowers of cactus leaves or cactus trees, and vegetables from the sea. Plant-based iron is also very helpful, such as dandelion, burdock and yellow dock. Dr. Sebi also stresses that you practice fasting, as fasting makes you eat less and recover faster. Another strong explanation why herpes can be healed by Dr. Sebi's diet is because the body gets rid of mucus. This is because the immune system becomes weak until the mucus membrane is weakened, and you get ill. For you to be protected, the mucus membrane has to stay healthy because it is your mucus membrane that is responsible for protecting the cells in your body. For treating herpes, the plant-based diets and herbs that are the key constituents of Dr. Sebi's alkaline cell foods are quite efficient. By detoxifying the bloodstream and efficiently nourishing the body, Dr. Sebi was able to treat herpes.

What Dr. Sebi used to treat herpes were the following steps:

- Put an end to eating foods containing acid. Ensure that the body should not feed on acidic ingredients.

- Flush your body of acids and toxins, and start eating herbs and alkaline diets that raise the oxygen content in your cells.

- Feed your body with the required nutrients at the cellular level that will restore, reconstruct, and totally reinforce your body.

- Fasting practice. During fasting, take herbs and water only. If fasting gets too hard for you, you should add green juice.

- Immediately after fasting, eat greens and fruits.

- Since the body has been rid of herpes, try to consume food from Dr. Sebi's dietary guide.

Detoxification is at the heart of the herpes virus's removal of the body- there is no other way to bring the requisite effects." Few information about Dr. Sebi's Herpes Cure Diet

The cure of herpes by Dr. Sebi Diet is rooted in certain reality. Let's look at some of the evidence that made Dr. Sebi's herpes treatment diet so successful. The Dr. Sebi diet is an alkaline diet focused on plants intended to eradicate acid from the body and to purify and detoxify the body effectively. The diet helps improve the immune system and helps the body fight against diseases such as the herpes virus. This diet helps remove mucus, repair a mucus membrane that is still weakened, and empowers your body to heal itself from diseases such as herpes.

The Dr. Sebi Diet Herpes Products

Five effective herbal products have been produced by Dr. Sebi that have helped many people to treat herpes. In order to treat herpes, these natural ingredients are what you need. The key ingredients used in Dr. Sebi's herpes drugs are below.

- Powder AHP Zinc

- Triphal

- Absolute Giloy tablet extract

- Mandoor of Punarnavadi

- AHP Powder Silver

Let us do a comprehensive overview of the components used in these items.

1. POWDER AHP ZINC

The word AHP stands for a distilled ayurvedic plant. Zinc purification is performed to produce AHP zinc powder with decoctions of natural herbs such as Aloe Vera. The strength of AHP zinc is a greater advantage than the normal zinc tablets you eat. AHP zinc powder is made from naturally occurring zinc, making it very convenient for the body to digest. AHP zinc powder also has the key characteristics of some of the herbs used in its preparation. Modern medicine also recognizes the value of zinc for herpes therapy, but instead of zinc capsules, it is safer to use AHP zinc powder. In treating herpes, AHP zinc powder is safer and more effective.

2. Triphal

Three excellent herbal combinations include Triphala. Harad, amla, baheda are the three herbs that make up Triphala. These three herbs have not only been recognised by Dr. Sebi for their efficacy, but other medicinal authorities have performed studies on these three excellent herbs and lauded their effectiveness. This blend of herbs is a good combination and can be used for both stable individuals and individuals with the herpes virus. This mixture of herbs will cleanse the body of unnecessary materials and contaminants, and also help purify the blood and certain organs in your body. Dr. Sebi not only prescribed this herbal mixture to his patients, but for maximum wellbeing and survival, he took it everyday.

3. Giloy Tablets Pure Extract

The Pure Extract Giloy tablets are manually produced from the highest quality Giloy extracts. The Giloy used to manufacture these tablets is derived from the Giloy with the highest quality. Dr. Sebi himself was a huge fan of Giloy, and today, modern medical scientists have agreed that Giloy can help the body fend off multiple diseases and even help improve fitness. Giloy is the best herb to strengthen your immunity and combat sexually transmitted diseases (STDs).

4. Mandoor of Punarnavadi

Punarnavadi mandoor is not a mineral purified from plants, but a balanced herbal mineral made from a mixture of herbs and minerals. An exceptional mix of good minerals such as calcium, iron, and wonderful herbs such as shunti, punarnava, alma, etc. Punarnavadi mandoor This mixture of herbal minerals acts perfectly on the liver and helps to kill liver toxins. This herbal mixture was prescribed to many of his patients by Dr. Sebi, and the explanation for this is that liver function was disrupted through illness, and Punarnavadi Mandoor is the best solution for getting liver function back to normal.

5. AHP Powder Silver

Ayurvedically herbo purified (AHP) is a procedure that involves purifying different minerals in herbal decoctions that make them usable for medicine. AHP ensures that the minerals not only preserve their outstanding abilities, but also extract the nutrients and characteristics of the herbs they are purified into. AHP powder, in particular your nervous system, is highly beneficial for your wellbeing. Dr. Sebi treated many of his patients with herpes with AHP silver powder, and the findings were still good. What makes herpes effective with AHP silver powder is that it acts on the nerves. The exact location where your body uses the herpes virus as its habitat and hiding place. By sending the silver nanoparticles into your nerves to eliminate and clear out the herpes virus in your neurons, AHP silver powder works.

Curing Herpes on a Budget with Dr. Sebi Diet

The method of treating herpes by Dr. Sebi is a simple method, and it is to nourish and detoxify the body. If you want to get rid of herpes in your body on a budget with this treatment, here are some of the stuff you need to do:

1. Fasting and Herbs

During the detoxification cycle, where you take in the requisite herbs alongside iron, the first thing you can do is to fast. Dr. Sebi has emphasized the value of iron with respect to healing on several occasions. This means that we should make use of the combination of green juices, water, and herbs for proper detoxification during this time.

2. Herbs and a diet of Alkaline

It is necessary to practice the Alkaline diet when pursuing the healing process for herpes. The alkaline diet is one where, with the limitation of meat and other starchy meals, you ingest vegetables and other basic meals. Dr. Sebi also emphasized the consumption of starch and meat as all that we ought to prevent while healing herpes. In order to help you remain on the Alkaline diet while treating your herpes, we also have a recipe list that you can follow. This implies that as you replenish the body and raise the immune system simultaneously, the body is washed of whatever may be battling the healing process.

Overall Review Guide

You can stop fried food as much as you can at this stage. Your diet will therefore take away all acid-forming ingredients. Hurry up while you get water and herbs. You will have to take fruits and vegetables as they enhance the healing process after you have finished your fast. If your herpes is gone, you will need to stay for a while with Dr. Sebi's recipes to keep you safe and make the healing process lasting. As we know from what we have heard from Dr. Sebi, herpes is curable, and it can be done on a budget as well. In order to have this done, you do not need to invest a lot, because all you have to do is follow the easy method highlighted here. You have to begin with the cleansing herbs to get Dr. Sebi herbs for herpes to function well for you.

Some of the cleansing herbs that you need to take are below:

Mullein

Mullein helps to cleanse the lungs and helps to activate the circulation of the lymph of the neck and chest.

Sarsaparilla Root

The root of Sarsaparilla helps to cleanse blood and target herpes. It is strongly recommended to use Jamaican sarsaparilla roots because it is a great iron source, and it is good for healing.

Dandelion

Dandelion allows the gallbladder and the kidney to cleanse.

Chaparral

Chaparral helps to cleanse the gallbladder and blood from toxic heavy metals and also to cleanse the lymphatic system.

Eucalyptuses

You should use eucalyptus in a sauna or steam to cleanse the hands.

Guaco Herb

Guaco treats wounds, cleanses the blood, encourages sweating, improves urination, makes the breathing system healthy, and improves digestion. Guaco leaves may be used for pain relief, prevention of some forms of venereal disease, phlegm expulsion, infection suppression, blood thinning, and bacterial death. When using the herb Guaco, you have to drink a lot of water.

Cilantro.

Cilantro helps extract from your cells heavy and toxic metals, and since the herpes virus hides behind your cell walls, this is important for herpes recovery.

Burdock Root

The Burdock root helps cleanse the liver and the lymphatic system.

Elderberry

Elderberry helps clear mucus from the upper respiratory tract and lungs.

Dr. Sebi Herbs for The Treatment of Herpes

Dandelion

A root plant that is particularly high in a chemical that helps to treat genital herpes is the Dandelion weed. In an attempt to minimize the influx of viruses into cells, the sap of the dandelion is externally added. The sap can be derived from either the root or the dandelion stalk. For a prolonged duration of 2 weeks, the removed sap must be rubbed on the genitals on a regular basis. If this procedure is taken religiously, the effects of herpes will only last for a few more days. The application routine is key to ridding the body of herpes symptoms after the sap. Using this drug for herpes, unlike a medical solution, has no side effects, no matter how long you take it.

BASIL

Of all the herpes anti-viral herbs found, this is simply one of the best. Basil leaves act like a magical treatment for herpes with their adaptogenic, infectious, antioxidant, immune-modulating, and analgesic powers. For certain other forms of medicines, basil is a common ingredient, but its effect on helping to rid the body of the herpes virus is less known. Basil leaves and their miraculous effects have supported people with allergies to a great degree. You'll require a batch of fresh basil leaves to get it correct for the natural herpes cure. These leaves should be boiled for a few minutes in a cup of water, after which you should drink the resultant liquid until it has cooled down. An excellent alternative to tea is this liquid leaf, too. And though you do not have an infection of herpes, this combination should be used regularly. During a herpes epidemic, though, make sure you take this herbal drink twice a day. For any given day, drinking this drink as much as you like would have no detrimental affect on your health.

Lavender oil

Through its antiseptic and regenerative qualities, Lavender essential oil is well regarded as a perfect natural treatment for herpes. A tiny bottle of lavender oil can be purchased off the shelves in every store. Lavender oil has an enticing scent that would do well to contrast with your cologne, unlike any other form of oil used in treating herpes. A cotton swab should be used on cold sores two to three times a day to spread the oil externally. Make sure that you wash your hands properly before and after applying the oil to prevent the bacteria from spreading to other places. You should add jojoba oil with it to form a mixture to make this natural herpes remedy more successful. Peppermint oil should also be considered in the mixture to further reinforce the effect. The most effective treatment for treating herpes has been found to be these three natural oils in a combination. The influence of oils will be hastened by the exceptional properties found in the combination of these oils. A cotton ball may be dipped in it for a gentle yet productive rub around cold sores after a suitable mixture has been developed. Wash the sore region with cold water after rubbing the covered cotton swab with essential oils over the cold sores, then dry the area with a dry cotton swab. During an epidemic of herpes, essential oil mixtures should be added twice a day to the appropriate regions.

Olive leaf extract

The herpes treatment with Olive Leaf Extract has been very successful. Olive leaves were crushed and used in drinks for patients in the early 80s, to alleviate fevers and malaria symptoms. Olives have also been used in the history of Moroccan medicine to balance blood sugar and regulate diabetes. There was no governing authority for the use of these leaves during all these years of early use and they performed miracles regardless. Today, numerous medical studies carried out on the olive leaves have provided promising findings all the way through the scrutiny of learned medical professionals. With several implementation approaches, olive leaves have proven to be special and promising. Now that the effectiveness of olive leaves has risen to scientific standards, now is your chance to try harvesting olive leaves to treat your herpes without delay or side effects.

How olive leaf extract eliminate herpes virus

Olive leaf extracts contain properties that, with the addition of the Herpes Zoster virus, are capable of removing viruses like HSV-1 and 2. The potent property described in extracts from olive leaves is none other than the compound of Oleuropein. In an olive plant, from the trunk to the leaves, this part is everywhere. The compound appears to be away from parasites and the plant defends itself. The major cause of the herpes epidemic has been found to be a lack of protein and stress. Basically, the herpes virus rises as the immune system weakens. What the olive leaf extract does in the body in an attempt to keep the herpes virus from breaking out is to provide a boost to the immune system. The olive leaf extracts tracks as taken into the bloodstream and attacks the bacteria within the body. The dead bacteria in the body are gotten rid of through natural detoxification. The less antigen the body has the better the risk of flare-ups being triggered by viruses and bacteria.

Why Your Best Choice is Dr. Sebi Herpes Cure

You already know by now what Dr. Sebi's treatment for herpes is all about. The explanation for this form of healing is not that a dollar is spent on an advertisement; rather, it is because of the way herpes victims have become captivated by their efficacy. The potency of De. The strategies and ideals of Sebi have made him the talk of the city and a revered hero among herpes sufferers. We're going to use this medium to convince you that the herpes cure of Dr. Sebi is the perfect alternative a patient with herpes can go for. Dr. Sebi was known for being a herbalist who cured a lot of people who had already lost hope of support. To make many individuals with incurable illnesses free of compensation, the herbalist clearly described the healing magic of herbs. The effect was unprecedented as well as unforeseen when the same theory was applied to herpes. Dr. Sebi was able to bring both of them under regulation, something scientists had been unable to treat for years. There was almost nothing operating on the cold sores and other herpes signs before Dr. Sebi came into the frame. This miracle herpes treatment will give another shot at life to any herpes patient. It is important to know how to use Dr. Sebi's cure; it is more important to understand that this conventional therapy is the best option around. We will go right through what this herpes treatment is made up of after this section is finished and dusted.

Why is Dr. Sebi the Perfect Treatment for Herpes?

It is best that it deals for herpes: from the point of view of efficacy, this is the best therapy so far. Around the world, there is very little reliable herpes care. Antiviral medications are available that are costly and unsuccessful. They just offer a false feeling of well-being when in fact, nothing in your body functions as it should. Despite some herpes patients' use of antiviral medications, the herpes simplex virus nevertheless thrives without any restrictions. Choosing antiviral medications over conventional narcotics is a lot of sacrifice as the former only mimics the signs of herpes and a lot of underlying side effects. Some other herbs are healthy but do not produce the same result as the cure of Dr. Sebi. This makes the cure of Dr. Sebi the only remedy that is suitable for a patient with herpes as nothing gets close to their curing prowess. It is the best choice and it is the only safe option: Dr. Sebi's solution is all-natural and every synthetic substance is devoid of all the ingredients found within. Since the very first man was created, herbs have been in existence and the reason why they are now favoured over traditional medicine is that they have zero side effects. Since Dr. Sebi's care consists exclusively of plants, you do not have to think about your actual and future health. These herbs, in truth, work like magic, not only to cure you from herpes, but also to improve your daily health. Those who have used Dr. Sebi's herpes remedy in the past have accepted the argument that after beginning the course, these herbs really improved their health as they became more energetic. This makes treating Dr. Sebi's herpes the only choice you can consider.

1. It's better that it's not cost-effective: you need a prescription for antiviral medications, Dr. Sebi herpes cure is different as when you make a buy you do not need that kind of prescription. A lot of the money that goes into consultation teaches you of this holistic medicine. Health is important, so it's exorbitant to waste money on antiviral medications, but that doesn't guarantee their efficacy. Dr. Sebi's herpes treatment is available on naturalherpescure.org, on the other hand. You should not have to pay a premium for consulting, because there are zero publicity expenses involved. You're paying only for what you get. You are not tossing out your hard-earned cash because this medicine is powerful and gets the job done.

2. It is better that it is certified by scientists: the argument of Dr. Sebi to treat herpes with herbs was confirmed by numerous medical and science tests to be authentic. More facts about the antiviral effects of the herbs used in the cure for herpes were contained in some of the tests. Without any side effects, normal antiviral properties are able to rid the body of the herpes virus. They have also been shown to be immune-modulatory, in addition to the antiviral properties found in these herbs. This means they improve the disease-fighting function of the body directly. In order for a

herpes patient to live a herpes free life, a better immune system essentially ensures that the replication of the herpes simplex virus should be kept under control. It is approved by all the studies on Dr. Sebi's herpes remedy as the perfect herpes treatment.

3. It's best because it gives you life free of herpes: the success of the cure for herpes by Dr. Sebi is the main reason why it is considered to be the best herpes treatment in the world. No other drug to heal herpes has been confirmed, only this one can. To live a herpes-free life, you need to trust Dr. Sebi's methods.

The points illustrated are some of the reasons why Dr. Sebi is the best treatment around for herpes. You should give this treatment a chance if you think it's time to bring an end to the pains herpes is taking you through. You need to know the content of this cure prior to that. Giloy is first and foremost. Because of its antipyretic properties, which match what is present in any antibiotic on the market, Giloy came to the fore. Scientists discovered years later that this herb relieves inflammation and increases immunity.

Revitalizing Herbs That Can Heal The Herpes Virus

Revitalizing herbs are herbs and oils which specifically target the herpes virus. After washing and detoxifying your body, it is crucial that you take these revitalizing herbs so that the herbs will clean your body entirely. The Dr. Sebi Herbs that will cure the herpes virus are below.

Pao Pereira

Pao Pereira helps to subdue the herpes virus successfully, and it also prevents the gene replication of the herpes virus. This herb is a wonderful herb that can help fight the herpes virus.

Pau d'Arco

Anti-viral effects against HSV-1 and HSV-2 and other viruses such as poliovirus, influenza, and vesicular stomatitis virus have been shown in vitro by the chemical constituents found in Pau d'Arco.

Oregano Essential Oil

A wonderful anti-viral that can kill the herpes virus is oregano essential oil. At ninety percent concentration, it performs best. As your lower spine is the place where HSV-2 is latent, add necessary oregano oil to your lower spine. You may even apply it under your tongue and into your genital region.

Ginger Essential Oil

Upon touch, the ginger essential oil can destroy the herpes virus. Although you should dilute the basic oil of ginger with carrier oil. The essential oil for ginger has the same influence as the essential oil for oregano.

Sea Salt Bath

Sea salt makes the skin absorb electrolysis which relieves the skin during an epidemic of the herpes virus. You need to apply a cup or half a cup of sea salt to a tub filled with warm water and soak the skin in it for some time to do this. Make sure the sea salt dissolves entirely.

Holy Basil

Stress is one of the reasons that by adrenal exhaustion, can cause a herpes outbreak. Holy basil is an adaptogen that relieves adrenal exhaustion by stress and prevents the spread of herpes.

How To Extract Essential Oils For Herpes

There are several herpes oils, and the one thing we have to take into account is the method of extraction. A delicate procedure that needs a lot of expertise as well as the right materials is the careful extraction of these oils from their natural sources. There are various methods of harvesting essential oils, but the two most important methods will be covered:

1. Steam distillation

2. Cold Press

Steam distillation

The steam distillation process makes use of steam and friction for the process of extraction. This method is an easy one, but it will certainly go wrong without the proper skills. The raw materials are put inside a stainless steel cooking oven, and it is broken down as the material is steamed, eliminating the explosive materials behind it. It travels up the chamber in gaseous form through the connecting tubing, which goes through the condenser, as the steam is freed from the plant. The gas returns to liquid form until the condenser is cold, and this is the critical oil that can be obtained from the water's surface.

Cold Pressing

The cold press operation removes oils from the citrus rind as well as the carrier oil of the seed oil. For the operation to go as expected, this process needs heat, but not as much heat as the steam distillation process with a maximum temperature of 120F. The object that is heated is put in a jar where a mechanism that rotates with thorns punctures it. The essential oils are released into a reservoir below the puncturing area until the puncturing process is complete. To extract the essential oil from the juice, these devices then use centrifugal energy. Both procedures are important, and with the right level of knowledge from professionals who know a lot about the process, if not a lot of harm, it must be handled correctly with the right level of information.

Other Aids this Alkaline diet targeted towards herpes will render

Reducing the possibility of stroke and hypertension

A big benefits of eating an alkaline diet is the reduction of a person's risk of stroke and hypertension. There is an anti-aging effect on a traditional alkaline diet. A robust outcome of the anti-aging results is that it dramatically decreases inflammation and promotes hormone development development. This has been shown to aid in maintaining cardiovascular health and to protect the body against typical health issues such as asthma, elevated cholesterol, stroke, kidney stones, and potential loss of memory.

Reduce systemic inflammation and discomfort

There is a link between diets that are alkaline and a dramatic decrease in chronic pain levels. The human health system is endangered by chronic acidosis. Which is the major cause of migraine, chronic back pain, pain in the joints, inflammation, signs of menstruation, and muscle spasms. For patients suffering from chronic pains, several studies demonstrate the health effects of an alkaline diet. A analysis carried out found that patients suffering from chronic back pain reported a substantial reduction in pain after alkaline-containing supplements were administered everyday for four weeks.

Give protection to bone density and muscle mass

In preserving and improving the bones in your body, bringing minerals into the body system plays a major role. Beyond the shadow of a doubt, evidence has shown that the more alkaline-rich fruits and vegetables you take on a daily basis, the better you are safe from the weakened bone muscle and strength known as Sarcopenia. When you take it, what an alkaline diet does is to better regulate the concentrations of the different nutrients required for bone-building and retaining a lean muscle mass in the body. Phosphate, magnesium and calcium are the nutrients that an alkaline diet balances. The increase in the development of vitamin D absorption and growth hormones is another advantage of an alkaline diet in this respect, which helps to better protect the bones and fight against many chronic diseases.

Weight loss

This diet wasn't made with weight loss in mind, but you can see weight loss because it is highly stringent. Often one of the key reasons that this diet is effective in losing weight is that it helps people avoid eating heavily caloric, oily, and sugary Western foods. Weight reduction comes as you drink less or equivalent quantities of calories than can be burned. You will get the dream body if you adopt this diet that is low in sugar, fat, and refined foods.

Enhances kidney function

The health of the kidneys is mainly affected by acidic diets and the structures inside the organ system are weakened. The pH of the urine mustn't be acidic to support kidney health. We will achieve this pH at which our kidneys stay safe and stable by eating a lot of alkaline food and eliminating acidic foods from our everyday routine. Alkaline diets have little effect on blood pH, but they may have a substantial influence on urine. Along with this diet, drinking a lot of water will help the kidneys even more. If you have some chronic kidney disease, so you should know that you are not the object of this diet. Since checking with the doctor first you will adopt the diet.

Reduces the risk of cancer

There are almost no relevant findings suggesting that an alkaline diet contributes to reduced cancer cases. Studies have shown, however, that if a person is to consume less meat and increase their intake of fresh fruits and vegetables, then that person is at a lower risk of cancer. Another research has found that having more vitamins in your diet, including vitamin C, would reduce cancer. In general, consuming more fruits and vegetables and eating fewer unhealthy and sugary foods contributes to a decline in cancer growth.

Reduces the risk of heart disease

Heart disease is the world's largest cause of death. It is mostly caused by consuming loads of fat and fatty ingredients, which contributes to plaque formation and artery blockage. The intake of fats in this diet declines dramatically, reducing the chances of contracting heart disease. Development hormones have since been found to be linked to reduced heart attack rates. An alkaline diet raises growth hormone levels, but it therefore reduces heart failure in conjunction.

Reduces the risk of muscle degradation

We tend to increase muscle loss as we get old or start using our muscles. A research published in 2013, however, found that individuals who adopt an alkaline diet could minimize muscle deterioration. The diet is poor in red meat, so there is a chance that muscle mass and strength will decrease.

Increases intestinal health

There is a list of nuts and seeds that you should consume on this diet with the inclusion of whole grains. It helps increase the consumption of fibre, which enhances the health of the small and large intestines. It helps to control daily bowel movements, and decreases the risk of certain diseases arising.

Decreases the harmful effects of processed foods

Increased sugar intake and fat content have been correlated with refined foods. They still produce plenty of calories, but their nutritional value is very low. If we specifically avoid artificial foods, certain chemicals and preservatives that serve no place in our bodies are removed from our diets.

It helps the brain

Not only is the growth hormone associated with a healthier cardiac condition, but it also helps to control the health of the mind. It is linked to an increase in cognition and memory. Consuming a nutritious diet high in fruits and vegetables helps in increased development of the brain.

It may improve back pain

Alkaline minerals are linked to the reduction of back pain, although it is yet to be determined if alkaline diets have the same effects. There is a fair probability that there will be similar consequences from the diet.

Decreases the level of inflammation

A great reduction of oxidative stress and inflammation is seen by diets high in fresh fruits and vegetables. This results in less pain and the creation of less infections in our bodies. They avoid magnesium deficiency and improve the absorption of vitamins. In the human body, magnesium plays an important role as an improvement in its amount is required for all the enzymes and processes in the human body to function properly.

Magnesium content deficiency can lead to headaches, nausea, cardiac issues, muscle pains, and sleep disorders. In activating vitamin D and preventing vitamin D deficiency, which is essential for the functioning of endocrine and general body immunity, magnesium is also required by the body.

Improving cancer protection and immune function

In disposing of waste or oxygenating the body, minerals are needed by the body. But the body struggles when there is a lack of the necessary minerals in the cells. Whenever there is a calcium deficiency in the body, vitamin absorption is zeroed out. Toxins and bacteria will also build up in the bloodstream, undermining the immune system in this manner. Although that can not happen for alkaline diets, as evidence has found that the death of cancerous cells occurs more with an alkaline body. Alkaline diets can help minimize inflammation and the future risks associated with diseases such as cancer that are harmful.

Help you in maintaining a healthy balanced weight

Not only can you limit the acid content of your body as you consume more alkaline foods, but you also shield the body from the dangers associated with obesity. This is likely since the amounts of Leptin and inflammation are lowered by alkaline diets, which have a direct impact on the appetite and fat-burning abilities.

Chapter eight: Fasting and Dr. Sebi diet

What Is Fasting?

The question on the lips of everyone is the safest way to fast safely. There is a need to paint a more straightforward image of what fasting is before we dive into that. For whatever excuse, absolute or partial abstinence from food is what is called fasting. The best juices are organic juices made from fresh fruits and vegetables from your blender, not from processed or frozen foods, according to Dr. Alvenia Fulton.

<u>Before you fast</u>

#1. The In order to properly cleanse the body, fasting comes in two steps. Second, before embarking on the real fasting, you must cleanse your body with natural herbs for at least five days.

2. #2. Your body will offer an indication of that when you are ready for the quick, and the indication you are going to get is during the process of cleansing with herbs. When you begin to feel hungry while cleansing, it's when you're really ready to start your soon. When your body is not ready, you should never fast, and if you are hungry after a fast, you should feed.

Why should you fast

If you try to learn how to correct the discomforts of your body, fasting will cure your body and keep you younger. The best fasting strategy is to clean the body until appetite is no longer there. You will fast as long as you want because there is no hunger. It will fade easily before your appetite returns. The tongue becomes white and soft; quickly until the tongue becomes red again and quickly until the sweetness of your breath and your body. Due to the elimination of all the radioactive waste in the body, the body can create its own fragrance.

What fasting will do

You'll look younger, feel younger, rejuvenate your face, and revitalize your hair and nails. In your body, fasting will do all these things. Your body will stay supple, full of energy, and shine with vitality if you fast. This is what we all want and nothing more than cleansing and fasting can do it. If not for fasting, nothing will do a better job of curing, growing, and relieving our body of waste and toxins (juice, vegetable, or water fasting).

What about Water fasting

It is safer to quick with water so it can rid the body of hazardous waste, cure the body of long-standing old dead cells. Cleansing the body and then beginning the bath immediately is the easiest way to achieve this. You will find that your skin becomes resonant, youthful and attractive as you fast.

Your hair, skin, and every gland in your body is going to respond to fasting. This is what they both need the deep cleansing from fasting that happens.

How to make preparations for fasting

Your fasting ought to start with cleansing. Before beginning your fast, use various natural herbs for 3 to 5 days, be it a drink, a vegetable, or swift water. To extract some of the poison and body waste, take herbs first. Most people have contaminants that have been in their bodies since they were infants, so before any form of fasting, herbs are really essential. For starters, the first day I tried fasting, I couldn't get up quickly enough to go to the bathroom on the 21st day because I had a lot of toxins flowing out of me.

How long should you fast?

You no longer feel exhausted, sluggish, or anxious and you feel young again after washing your body with herbs, easily for 21 or 30 days until you no longer have a 'coated' tongue. You are going to be asked by the people around you what you are doing; you would look more young. Then, crack the fast and begin again; you don't need to take medications to do what you want if you cleanse the body easily and properly. Male or female, your sex drive will continue to work well and if they are cleansed and quick, your hormones will work.

Fast to Cleanse Toxins

You will come to the conclusion that food isn't what keeps us alive as humans. What makes us alive, in our bodies, is getting rid of toxins and pollution. When we eat what nature has given us and on top of that, we immediately cleanse our bodies, our body and mind will change. Our fathers, including the young men of today, do not have issues with prostate glands. Our grandmothers, too have not lost their youthful factor, as it is in the world of today. As a matter of fact, at the age of 49, my great grandma had twin boys, but considering all the medical discoveries, this is unheard of in the 21st century. We will remain well, live longer, and all pain in the body will disappear as we feed according to what nature has in store for us. Ultimately, good health will prevail as we cleanse our bodies and adhere to the right diet.

How do you break your fast?

Exactly the way you began, you have to break a fast. I say, by this, get a juice, boil it up and take it for five consecutive days. You're going to have more resources than you need. You're not going to be famished. If after an extended fasting time, you move back into taking steaks, you will get sick. That diet is going to make you fall sick. As they induce body pain and ache, you have to completely avoid all those forms of food. You didn't come to this planet for a fleeting life to live. There are so many different ways of fasting. The aim of this guide and knowledge is to know the best way for you to fast. Ultimately, all this is about choosing a form of fasting that fits best for you.

Foods When Fasting

Dr. Sebi has suggested easy-to-digest foods and ones that can drive the efficiency of the body to its best. Fasting is essentially abstinence from food, and this act significantly increases the separation from the body of waste materials. Both types of stuff we take that can diminish our physical wellbeing are pollutants, chemical contaminants, synthetic drugs, electrical radiation. Fasting is a process that eliminates from the body contaminants such as mucus, fecal matter, parasites, and phlegm rapidly.

What type of food to prepare for fasting

Dr. Sebi, the world-renowned scientist, advises that if you have to eat for medical purposes during a fast, you need to know the best combinations of food to eat that will further help to remove waste and toxins. Eating natural alkaline fruits, vegetables, and freshly produced juices from these fruits is more beneficial.

#1 There is a need to consume foods that are rich in minerals that can be quickly broken down and digested by the body to provide the elements the body requires during a fast. Before starting the healing process, this diet will ensure that the body has excess energy to remove waste materials.

Checklist for Dr. Sebi Fasting Foods

Here are the advantages of the fasting food of Dr. Sebi; here are the benefits to the body when you consume the fasting foods prescribed. All natural foods contain 92 minerals contained in the earth's soil, 27 of which are found in the human body and play an important role in preserving good health and getting our body back to its original state of health. These foods contain the following advantages that are important to the body's optimum and proper functioning.

The fasting foods also provide:

Alkalinity

Iron, calcium, magnesium, copper, zinc, and many other minerals

Expel mucus

Easy to digest, assimilate, and used by the body

They flush out the body and detox harmful wastes

Neutralize the body's PH balance

Restore the body overall good health

Get rid of toxins

The Fasting Eating Foods

Fruits:

- Seeded melons

- Mangoes

- All kinds of berries

- Papaya and many more

During fasting, Vegetables to Eat

For medical purposes or some other condition you are in, whether you have to feed during your fast. Because of their capacity to help the body remove mucus or toxins due to their high mineral content, these vegetables are suitable for consumption:

- Dandelion leaves

- Green leafy vegetables

- Kale

Downsides of the Dr. Sebi Diet

Although the diet of Dr. Sebi is really beneficial in increasing one's health and may enhance people's quality of life, there may be a few downsides or drawbacks of adopting the diet of Dr. Sebi to the letter.

Restricted food intake

A modified vegan diet with supplement requirements, in nature, is the Dr. Sebi diet. However while vegan diets tend to be very stringent too the diet of Dr. Sebi goes much further and has a lot more constraints. Not only are adherents expected to exclude animal products outright and focus solely on plant-based diets, such as most vegans, but more stringent restrictions are also in effect. For starters, traditional vegan diets permit any fruit and merely set restrictions on the amount of consumption. However the diet of Dr. Sebi goes as far as banning us from consuming certain kinds of food, such as Roma tomatoes or beefsteak tomatoes, while cherry and plum tomatoes are allowed. This will lead to some challenges in adhering to the diet, as it has been found that it is harder to adopt rigid diets. As such if one finds it difficult or impractical to adopt the diet, they would not be able to gain in the first place from the diet, undermining the diet's intent.

Reliance on Supplementation

Although vitamins are not an intrinsically negative thing, based on where one is in the country, the Dr. Sebi diet allows one to take various types of supplements, which can be pricey or difficult to source. Dr. Sebi's dietary supplements are essential, but not exclusive, which ensures that other supplements can still be used to compensate for any vitamin shortages that could have arisen along the way. This suggests that one may be unsure as to what additional supplements may be needed, and therefore one who wishes to start the diet of Dr. Sebi may contact a nutritionist to devise their diet plan in compliance with the rules of Dr. Sebi and to figure out what additional supplements may be appropriate, if any. Furthermore the fact that these nutrients inevitably expose the fundamental weakness of a vegan-based diet, where only plant-based items are used, adds to nutritional deficits that need to be accounted for by supplementation. For starters, in vegan diets and even more so in the more conservative form of Dr. Sebi, protein appears to be difficult to come by and protein is an important macronutrient for us to remain healthy. While nuts are a protein source, consuming all the protein we need only by nut intake, and hence the need for supplementation, seems to be hard and impractical. Nutrients such as omega 3, iron, calcium and vitamin B12 are other foods that need to be supplemented, both of which are essential to keep the body healthy and safe, but can be difficult to come by while adopting the diet of Dr. Sebi, and therefore need supplements.

Risk Of Vitamin Deficiencies

One very important thing we need to note is that while vegetables are highly nutrient-dense, few of the essential nutrients are only the best sources. There are certain nutrients that can not be produced by an all-plant-matter diet, such as vitamin B-12, vitamin D, calcium, and some fatty acids such as the long-chain Omega-3 fatty acid typically found in fish, since the body can not produce these nutrients using the building blocks it obtains from fruit, but rather must be found in fish As such, using adequate supplementation, vegans are advised to supplement their diet to ensure that they get all the required nutrients to preserve their health and to ensure that they maintain a healthy diet. While supplements are crucial in the Dr. Sebi diet and are used in the diet plan, food portions and meal design are not defined by the diet itself which means that the supplements may not be enough to substitute for nutritional deficits that may exist. Because the diet of Dr. Sebi does not actually recommend what to consume exactly and instead prescribes what should be ingested, certain persons can eat more of one item and less of another, which may contribute to nutritional imbalances, even with the addition of the supplements required. For instance, one instance of this will be B-12 nutritional deficiency. Many who are primarily vegetarian or vegan and do not drink animal products are already at risk of having a shortage of vitamin B-12, and are thus urged to take vitamins to mask it. The diet supplements of Dr. Sebi does not contain enough B-12 vitamins that one requires, and this is not completely obvious, since the diet supplements of Dr. Sebi are essential, but not exclusive, implying that other supplements should still be used to compensate for any vitamin shortages that may have arisen along the way. One of run the risk of developing deficiencies without consulting a trained nutritionist, and so special caution should be taken while preparing and designing a diet plan around the diet principles of Dr. Sebi. Meat, like in any other vegan diet, protein appears to be in low supply and can be covered for by supplements, is another nutrient that can be looked out for by those who take the Dr. Sebi diet.

Foods to eat

The Dr. Sebi diet is very strict as to what foods are permitted and what foods are not allowed or what can be avoided, as discussed earlier. This list could be very detailed, and it will have to be addressed here as such. The following will be those basic items included on a diet:

Fruits

Under the Dr. Sebi diet, not all fruits are required, and fruits that are permissible will be apples, currants, dates, elderberries, grapes, peaches, pears, key seeded limes, figs, cantaloupe, mangoes, melons, prickly pears, and tamarinds. Notably, non-seeded fruit varieties are not included in this list, since this would include the use of manipulated foods that Dr. Sebi was unable to examine, and they should be avoided, considering the unpredictable results.

Vegetables

Similarly, under the Dr. Sebi diet, not all vegetables are required to be eaten, and the list of vegetables allowed is as follows: avocado, cactus flowers, chickpeas, lettuce (NOT iceberg lettuce), kale, bell peppers, cucumber, mushrooms (NOT shiitake), okra, sea vegetables, olives, squash, tomatoes (cherry and plum tomatoes ONLY), zucchini. Take notice of the exceptions mentioned, such as not consuming iceberg lettuce, and cherry and plum are the only tomato variants authorized.

Grains

The grains permissible are Fonio, Khorasan wheat, rye, wild rice, quinoa, spelt, amaranth. Notice that whole grains are encouraged here and the particular variant of wheat that is encouraged is Kamut, or Khorasan wheat. It should also be remembered that the grains here which take the form of pasta, bread, flour or cereal, but leavened food is forbidden and foods prepared with baking powder or yeast are not allowed.

Nuts, Seeds, and Oils

The nuts, seeds, and oils permitted under the Dr. Sebi diet are avocado oil, coconut oil (unprocessed), grape seed oil, Brazilian nuts, hemp seeds, raw sesame seeds, raw tahini butter, walnuts, hemp seed oil, olive oil (virgin/unprocessed), sesame oil. Note that as the refined oil version is prohibited, non-processed oils are permissible.

Herbs and Spices

While the diet of Dr. Sebi promotes, and practically demands water intake, at least one gallon a day, herbal teas are tolerated. Herbal teas are all permitted, such as elderberry, fennel, tila, ginger, burdock, mango, tila, fennel and chamomile. Herbs and spices are also approved, including oregano, basil, bay leaf, dill, basil, achiote, habanero, cayenne, onions, estragon, garlic, ginger, sea salt, thyme, seaweed, agave syrup and date sugar. And if one has a sweet tooth, this allows one to produce delicious and satisfying foods, as agave syrup and date sugar are permitted, while white sugar and cane sugar are not allowed.

Facts to prevent potential complications, you should read about the alkaline diet

With dietitians and the health-conscious, alkaline diet is becoming more and more normal. It should not be surprising that this diet is effective in helping the body to sustain its peak fitness, maximize its resilience and achieve overall well-being. Nevertheless, like many other diets, the Alkaline Diet still has its share of risks. We're showing you three of the main risks, but you can't slip into this diet.

1. Eating all alkaline foods alone will not be safe. Other types and quantities of acidic compounds are also needed by the body. Other foods that contain the nutrition the body needs are recommended in order to stay balanced.

2. The nutrients needed for optimum health are not met by the alkalization of the diet. Nutrients such as omega-3 and other main fatty acids are not produced by alkaline diets. Of course, everyone with health consciousness knows that except for meat and dairy products, he or she needs the nutrients of any food type. Foods that provide the body with acid minerals and alkaline minerals are also essential to consume.

3. Toxic products include leather and rubber. You still eat poisonous toxin residue or residues whether you consume water or food from a plastic bottle. When you eat plastic-stocked milk, that is also true. This is one thing you need to acknowledge. For almost all that impacts and enters our bodies with all sorts of chemicals, the body is fragile.

When you buy alkaline products from the internet, check that the source is real. To ensure that you have the proper ph level, it is therefore equally important to have a PH control package. When slightly finished, alkalizing the food would be good.

Conclusion

The diet approved by Dr. Sebi, also known as Alfredo Bowman, has certified some 100% vegan food products that are not refined or changed. Dr. Sebi is not a doctor or may not hold a degree, but he appears to be a herbalist who is self-taught. However, disorders such as coronary failure, diabetes, kidney dysfunction or liver disease may be avoided by following this diet. It is also possible to use this diet to lose weight and reverse or avoid the health conditions already listed. Although it has few drawbacks, detoxification and cleaning have some health advantages. Few of the benefits of this are that it keeps you healthy and physically fit, increases digestion, improves the individual's concentration. Other than that, natural detoxification procedures such as dry cleaning, cupping, souping, exercise etc are also available. By changing this diet, shinier hair, healthier and clean skin, increased immune and overall optimum health may have many health benefits. Herbs and Food Recipe promises the diversity and versatility of the person who looks forward to adopting Dr. Sebi's accepted diet. For the accepted pieces, there are tons of variations that can be accomplished and enjoyed. Dr Sebi developed his advanced diets with his wealth of expertise as an expert in natural health and wellness. Fruits with nuts, agave syrup, wild rice, coconut oil, olive oil, and many more are part of his diet. He went on to develop his own basic six food classes, which are; Dead, Raw, Live, Medicines, Hybrid, and Modified Genetically. Dead Food is a meal that can last for days without going sour. Some examples are fruit chips, flavored crackers, flavored foods, and meal replacement bars, which are highly refined, synthesized, and less nutritious. This food category is very prevalent because it is fast, tasty and easy, but it includes additives, flavors and artificial colors, and unknown ingredients. The intake of such foods leads to diseases such as diabetes, stroke, heart disease, and obesity, etc. Chemically modified and refined foods have now been detected to be key players in inducing inflammation of the body. It induces chronic inflammation as these dead foods accumulate in the body, which results in weight gain, higher blood pressure, arthritis, and high blood sugar levels, etc. All the effects of the body responding to these dead foods are headaches, aches, brain fog, chemical imbalance, bad sleep. It's going to be an attempt to start dismantling herpes stigmas. The concern with the wellbeing problem with herpes is that the suffering inflicted on people with the infection causes entirely needless mental problems. The stigma impacts both physical and mental health, and remains a significant concern.

The diet recommends eating a decent amount of food, vitamins, nutrients, including vegetables and fruit, and plant compounds. Decreased inflammation and oxidative stress and defense from certain diseases have been linked with diets rich in fruits and vegetables. The rate of cancer and heart disease was 25 percent and 31 percent lower for a survey of 65,226 persons consumed seven or more servings of vegetables and fruit per day. Most individuals, though don't eat enough food. In a 2017 study, the criteria for fruit and vegetables were fulfilled by 9.3% and 12.2% of the population respectively. The diet of Dr Sebi also advocates the intake of fibre-rich whole grains and good fats, including almonds, seeds and plant oils. A decreased risk of heart attack is associated with such goods. Ultimately, diets that limit ultra-processed foods provide a higher average diet. Dr Sebi's diet emphasizes nutrient-rich foods that reduce the risk of heart disease, cancer and inflammation, such as vegetables, bananas, whole grains and healthy fats.

www.ingramcontent.com/pod-product-compliance
Lightning Source LLC
Chambersburg PA
CBHW072030230526
45466CB00020B/1203